Pulmonary Rehabilitation
An Interdisciplinary Approach

Pulmonary Rehabilitation

An Interdisciplinary Approach

Edited by

Rachel Garrod PhD, MSc, MCSP
St George's Hospital Medical School
and Kingston University, London

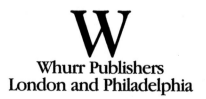

Whurr Publishers
London and Philadelphia

© 2004 Whurr Publishers Ltd
First published 2004
by Whurr Publishers Ltd
19b Compton Terrace
London N1 2UN
England

British Library Cataloguing in Publication Data

A catalogue record for this book is available from the
British Library.

ISBN 1 86156 421 X

Contents

Preface   vii

Contributors   ix

Chapter 1   Disability and handicap in COPD   1
                R. Garrod

Chapter 2   Selection of patients: who benefits?   11
                M. Decramer, R. Gosselink, T. Troosters

Chapter 3   Health-related quality of life and
                pulmonary rehabilitation   22
                J. Bestall

Chapter 4   Exercise prescription and training   36
                C. Clark, L. Cochrane, S. Conroy

Chapter 5   Assessment of exercise performance and
                muscle function in pulmonary rehabilitation   54
                R. Gosselink, T. Troosters, M. Decramer

Chapter 6   COPD: a biopsychosocial approach   78
                M. Fitzpatrick, J. Fearn

Chapter 7   Nursing and respiratory care at home   96
                J. Scullion

Chapter 8   Occupational therapy in pulmonary rehabilitation   114
                P. J. Turner-Lawlor

Chapter 9 Physiotherapy and the management of dyspnoea   **138**
              R. Garrod

Chapter 10 Dietary management of COPD   **154**
              E. Wouters, A. Schols, M. Vermeeren

Chapter 11 Cost-effectiveness of pulmonary rehabilitation   **173**
              T. Griffiths

Chapter 12 Future prospects for pulmonary rehabilitation   **187**
              P. M. A. Calverley

Index   **195**

Preface

As a researcher and a physiotherapist involved in the clinical delivery of services for patients with chronic obstructive pulmonary disease, I have been passionate about pulmonary rehabilitation for a number of years. Why am I so passionate about this service? I think because pulmonary rehabilitation has been the first vehicle for delivery of an integrated pathway of holistic care that truly attempts to address patients' needs. Pulmonary rehabilitation works, we know that; there is strong evidence to prove it has beneficial effects on exercise tolerance, muscle strength and, potentially, exacerbations. But, more importantly, we know it benefits sufferers by improvements in their ability to perform daily activities, a reduction in the perception of breathlessness and improvements in health-related quality of life (HRQoL). These can be monumental improvements for many patients, making real differences to their lives.

Pulmonary rehabilitation can help patients cope with their disability better, can help them tolerate their disease condition better, and can help them manage it better. It is concerned with enabling patients to make choices in their lives concerning their health. As health care professionals, we play a crucial role in facilitating empowerment; however, this means we face some significant challenges. We must ensure that all patients have access to appropriate rehabilitation care and that we define that care for all. We must endeavour to fully identify and address individual needs; and we must encourage lifelong behavioural change. But, most importantly, we must help the patient feel equipped to make this change. These are not easy challenges, and we shall not achieve them when working in isolation. The aim of this book is to help health care professionals identify and successfully meet these challenges.

This book is a collaborative work with chapters from well-known experts in the field, both in practical delivery and in research. The research base for pulmonary rehabilitation is significant and growing daily and the chapters in this book reflect the important contribution of this research to our understanding of the components of successful rehabilitation. We have attempted to synthesize and analyse the literature to enable the reader to make evidence-based decisions concerning a number of germane issues.

Pulmonary Rehabilitation: An Interdisciplinary Approach is an integrated evaluation of the effect of pulmonary rehabilitation on patient care, with critical assessment of outcome tools and the important contribution of an interdisciplinary approach.

Rachel Garrod
July 2004

Contributors

Janine Bestall PhD, BSc
Academic Unit of Palliative Medicine, Royal Hallamshire Hospital, Sheffield

Peter Calverley PhD
Clinical Science Centre, University Hospital Aintree, Liverpool

Chris Clark BSc, BA, MD, FRCP
Clinical Senior Lecturer in Medicine, University of Glasgow and Consultant Physician, Hairmyers Hospital, Glasgow

L M Cochrane MB, ChB, MD
Clinical Psychologist, Hairmyers Hospital, Glasgow

Sarah Conroy BSc MCSP
Senior 1 Physiotherapist, Hairmyers Hospital, Glasgow

Marc Decramer MD, PhD
Professor of Medicine, Respiratory Division, University Hospitals Leuven, Belgium

Jacqueline Fearn BSc, DClinPsych
Chartered Clinical Psychologist, South Devon Healthcare Trust

Maureen Fitzpatrick BEd, BSc, DClinPsych
Consultant Clinical Psychologist, South Devon Healthcare Trust

Rachel Garrod PhD, MSc, MCSP
Senior Lecturer, School of Physiotherapy, St George's Hospital Medical School, London

Rik Gosselink PT, PhD
Respiratory Rehabilitation and Respiratory Division, University Hospitals
Leuven, Belgium

Tim Griffiths PhD, FRCP
Section of Respiratory Medicine, University of Wales College of
Medicine, Penarth, Vale of Glamorgan

Anna Maria Schols PhD
Associate Professor, Department of Respiratory Medicine, University
Hospital Maastricht, The Netherlands

Jane Scullion RGN, MSc
Nurse Consultant and part-time Clinical Fellow, Respiratory Unit, UHL
Glenfield Leicester, Department of General Practice and Primary Care,
University of Aberdeen

Thierry Troosters PT, PhD
Respiratory Rehabilitation and Respiratory Division, University Hospitals
Leuven, Belgium

Patricia Turner-Lawlor DipCOT, SROT, MBAOT
Research Occupational Therapist, Pulmonary Rehabilitation, Department
of Respiratory Medicine, Vale of Glamorgan

Maria Adriana Vermeeren BSc
Department of Dietetics, University Hospital Maastricht,
The Netherlands

Emile Wouters MD, PhD
Professor in Respiratory Medicine, University Hospital Maastricht,
The Netherlands

Chapter 1
Disability and handicap in COPD

R. GARROD

Pulmonary rehabilitation in context

Physical exercise and chest-wall expansion was first introduced by Charles Dennison in 1895 in *Exercise for Pulmonary Invalids*. By the twentieth century, Dr Alvan Barach of New York, while investigating dyspnoea, discovered that the 'lean-forward position' improved the perception of breathlessness. Investigations began into the role of breathing exercises on exercise tolerance (Barach 1974). Later work confirmed these findings (Sharp et al. 1980). In 1966, research into pulmonary rehabilitation was instigated in Denver and Minneapolis, USA, by Thomas Petty and co-workers (Petty 1968). The intention of their study was to evaluate the outcome of what was termed 'comprehensive and rehabilitative care'. Interest was sustained and refocused in the late 1980s when Brian Make wrote a review article in which he discusses the role of occupational and physiotherapeutic interventions and identified the gains that may be demonstrated after pulmonary rehabilitation (Make 1986). Pulmonary rehabilitation has continued to gain credence in Britain since then, and much work has been achieved in the development of sensitive and reliable outcome measures. Research and scientific work has been rigorous, and a number of working parties and international bodies have defined pulmonary rehabilitation and provided guidelines for the administration of the service (Anonymous 1997, Anonymous 1995, Morgan et al. 2001, Morey 2000). Pulmonary rehabilitation is a holistic therapy provided to patients with respiratory disease that aims to address both the psychological and physical problems associated with chronic respiratory disease. Although there is much work supporting the role of this multidisciplinary therapy, a recent press release by the British Thoracic Society has highlighted the urgent need for increased rehabilitation services in patients such that 'the lives of at least 600,000 patients, mostly with chronic obstructive pulmonary disease, would be improved by access to rehabilitation' (BTS website). In an earlier review article considering cost-effectiveness it was concluded that pulmonary rehabilitation 'is likely to result in financial benefits to the health service' (Griffiths et al. 2001).

An executive report commissioned by the Research and Development Directorate of the National Health Service was published in 1999 suggesting government interest in the provision of pulmonary rehabilitation. The report supported the view that hospital-based outpatient pulmonary rehabilitation programmes were effective in improving quality of life and exercise tolerance, although at the time of publication there were few data concerning long-term effectiveness, cost evaluation or selection criteria. The committee noted that 'there is likely to be increasing demand for such services in the future'.

Definitions

An early definition of pulmonary rehabilitation was devised by the Pulmonary Rehabilitation Committee of the American College of Chest Physicians. In 1981, they described pulmonary rehabilitation as:

> an art of medical science wherein an individually tailored multidisciplinary programme is formulated which, through accurate diagnosis, therapy, emotional support and education, stabilises or reverses both the physiology and psycho-pathology of pulmonary disease and attempts to restore the patient to the highest possible functional level allowed by his pulmonary handicap and overall life situation. (Hodgkin et al. 1982)

A number of changes and research developments led by specialists in the field have necessitated revision and adaptation of the original definition. A pulmonary rehabilitation workshop was commissioned by the National Institutes of Health (NIH), and in 1994 this working party published a new definition:

> Pulmonary rehabilitation is a multidisciplinary continuum of services directed to persons with pulmonary disease and their families, usually by an interdisciplinary team of specialists, with the goal of achieving and maintaining the individual's maximum level of independence and functioning in the community. (Cole and Fishman 1994)

The more recent definition explicitly states that the goal of pulmonary rehabilitation is to achieve and maintain 'independence and functioning in the community'. Greater recognition is made of the role families play in the management of the disease and the need for interdisciplinary working. Thus, health care professionals must not merely work side by side in the provision of rehabilitation but ensure that an integrated programme is delivered where members complement but do not duplicate roles.

Rationale for holistic programme

A wide contextual framework is required in order to fully appreciate the complex nature of respiratory disease and its effects on the sufferer. The World Health Organization has previously identified three dimensions of disease as, 'impairment, disability and handicap'; however, a new revision of its International Classification of Functioning (ICF) has recently been undertaken (Figure 1.1). This ensures a more positive outlook and better reflects the complexity of problems faced by patients with a health condition (World Health Organization 2001). ICF now defines function by describing the dimensions as body functions and structure, activity and participation. With respect to patients with pulmonary disease, body functions and structure will include the respiratory and cardiovascular systems, the musculature (peripheral and respiratory) and skeletal systems, and the brain and co-ordinating centres. It is important to remember that problems at the level of the body, termed 'impairments', are not confined to the respiratory system.

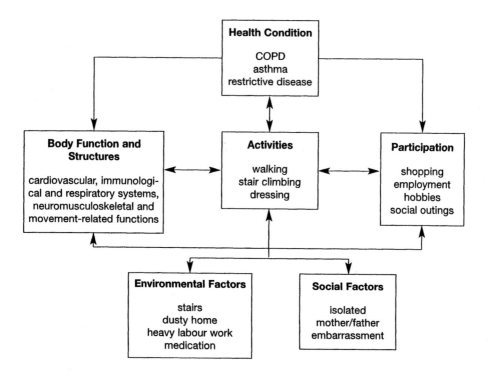

Figure 1.1 International Classification of Functioning, Disease and Health (ICF): application to respiratory disease.

Function at the level of the individual is now termed 'activity' rather than 'disability'. This reinforces the positive aspects of an individual's performance; patients with respiratory disease may experience 'limitations in activity', while other activities may still be performed, albeit with difficulty. The purpose of pulmonary rehabilitation is to emphasize and maximize activities as well as enabling the individual to participate at a social and environmental level. Participation is the most complex aspect of function, since it is affected by the interplay of the health condition, the body and structures and activities within the context of an individual's life and society. Effective therapy for the individual requires an understanding of all these dimensions and a combined holistic approach which comprehensively addresses the needs of the individual.

Body function and structure

There are many texts that document the pathophysiological process underlying respiratory disease, and chronic obstructive pulmonary disease in particular. It is not the purpose of this book to reiterate these phenomena. However, airflow obstruction and associated hyperinflation result in a number of distressing symptoms, the predominant being that of dyspnoea. Inflammatory processes common in respiratory disease have damaging effects on the peripheral musculature and contribute to worsening airflow obstruction (Agusti et al. 2003). As such, it is essential that patients admitted to pulmonary rehabilitation programmes undergo optimization of medical therapy and pharmacological therapy. These may include oxygen, non-invasive ventilation and steroid administration. Thorough assessment is the key to effective pulmonary rehabilitation, and, although rehabilitation is unlikely to affect measures of airflow obstruction such as FEV_1, full spirometry assessment is recommended to enable accurate classification of patients and record changes over time as a result of worsening pathology (BTS 2001). More extensive lung-function tests may help identify those patients who will achieve most from rehabilitation and those patients for whom adjunctive techniques may be required. There is evidence to suggest that general body exercise training may result in improvements in respiratory muscle strength, highlighting the importance of assessment of respiratory muscle strength (O'Donnell et al. 1998a). Moreover, hyperinflation is associated with increased breathlessness and may prove to be a more sensitive measure of change after rehabilitation (O'Donnell et al. 1998a).

Leg fatigue is often reported as a factor limiting exercise in patients with COPD (Hamilton et al. 1995), and muscle weakness is a significant contributor to impaired-exercise performance (Gosselink et al. 1996). Indeed, leg fatigue is experienced at lower work intensities in COPD patients compared with normal subjects, and dysfunction may be responsible for the early onset of lactic acidosis (Maltais et al. 1998). Whittom and co-workers from Canada (Whittom et al. 1998) have identified histochemical and morphological differences in the quadriceps muscles of patients with COPD compared with normal age-matched subjects, and Bernard et al. (Bernard et al. 1998) showed an association between the degree of airflow obstruction and the strength of the quadriceps. Important studies of peripheral muscle characteristics have reported on biopsies taken from vastus lateralis and demonstrate a reduction in oxidative enzymes compared with healthy individuals. These studies have shown that training can improve the mitochondrial content of these enzymes, associated with changes in endurance and reduction in lactic acidosis (Maltais et al. 1996). Strength may be reduced as a result of inactivity or possibly as an effect of worsening inflammatory processes. Further chapters in this text will address specific issues of assessment and exercise training in respiratory disease.

Activity limitation

There is much work documenting limitation in activity in COPD. In 2000, a British Lung Foundation survey reported that 75 per cent of patients with COPD had difficulty gardening, and 79 per cent said they found climbing stairs difficult. In addition to this, over 50 per cent of patients described themselves as severely or moderately short of breath during routine daily activities, such as dressing and washing (Garrod et al. 2000). Assessment of activities of daily living, of desired goals and health-related quality of life enable personnel within rehabilitation programmes to focus and maximize activities and participation.

Characteristics of rehabilitation programmes

Thus, in order to address the myriad problems for respiratory patients, pulmonary rehabilitation programmes must incorporate a number of features. There is strong evidence to support the role of exercise training aimed at increasing peripheral muscle strength and endurance (Lacasse et al. 1997). The aim of rehabilitation is to improve functional limitations, thus necessitating a component of functional training. Nutritional imbalance should be identified and interventions considered. Strategies to minimize dyspnoea and reduce the work of breathing must be implemented and reinforced throughout training. Psychosocial issues require identification and management, and can be successfully implemented as part of, or in conjunction with, the rehabilitation process. For different patient groups, adjuncts such as respiratory muscle training, non-invasive ventilation or supplemental oxygen may be required. Pulmonary rehabilitation requires active participation from the recipients of the intervention and, as such, an educational component to the programme is recommended. This should be integrated with and built on the physical aspects of the programme. These themes are further developed within the chapters of this book.

The aims of pulmonary rehabilitation are to:

- reduce dyspnoea
- increase exercise tolerance
- improve functional performance
- increase muscle endurance (peripheral and respiratory)
- improve muscle strength (peripheral and respiratory)
- ensure long-term commitment to exercise
- help allay patient fear and anxiety
- increase knowledge of lung condition and promote self-management.

The multidisciplinary team approach

Pulmonary rehabilitation is 'a multidisciplinary continuum of services' (Cole and Fishman 1994), and, in order to effectively manage the problems outlined, a team approach is required. However, evidence is lacking concerning staffing requirements, and, although guidelines recommend a multidisciplinary approach, they are often not explicit concerning precise roles (BTS 2001). Much will depend upon local resources. Indeed, collaboration between different disciplines is required at the implementation stage, before delivery even begins.

The members of that team may consist of a number of health care professionals – physiotherapists and occupational therapists, respiratory nurses, doctors, lung-function technicians, dieticians, clinical psychologists working together – and liaison with social services and community teams. Although there may appear to be an overlap between the roles, it is essential that the team works together to provide an integrated service; the omission of one member can lead to inappropriate management, inadequacy of assessment and a disjointed approach to delivery. The physiotherapist may supervise and deliver the exercise programme; however, cognitive-behavioural therapy in conjunction with training may result in greater benefits than training alone (Toevs et al. 1984). Pacing exercise and daily activities help to conserve energy, enabling the patient to perform more effectively. A combined delivery of occupational therapy and physiotherapy can enhance the training experience. Good access to medical support ensures patients optimize medication and more effectively manage exacerbations. The ready availability of medical personnel during the rehabilitation period may significantly reduce hospitalizations. Respiratory nurses from primary care may be involved in integrating patients with milder disease, in education and support, and in the referral process. Good respiratory technician support will ensure adequate characterization of the patients and may be used to monitor progress and maintenance. Nutritional intervention is often undervalued, and although evidence is yet to be produced to support the role of nutritional supplements, we know that mortality is independently associated with malnourishment and respiratory muscle weakness (Schols et al. 1998).

Liaison with community services will help enhance long-term behavioural change and perhaps identify further appropriate interventions for patients with severe limitations in activity.

At present, when we think of pulmonary rehabilitation programmes, we tend to associate them with outpatient hospital-based programmes. Yet the demand for rehabilitation is increasing, individual patient needs are different, and access may prove problematic for many patients. Pulmonary rehabilitation works in all settings, given that the intensity, duration and frequency of the programme are adequate. However, research trials have highlighted a few relevant issues. Home-based training may be effective, although a number of home-individualized programmes have shown little benefit or only small changes (Wedzicha et al. 1998, Busch and McClements 1988, McGavin et al. 1977). In a more recent randomized controlled trial of 60 COPD patients, there was no benefit of home-based training on maximal walking distance or cycle ergometry; however, there was a doubling in sub-maximal walking intensity (Hernandez et al. 2000). While this improvement is not to be underestimated, it is likely to be mainly due to practice effects, since the walking test itself featured prominently in the training schedule. Training was performed at a designated area near the patient's home and consisted of walking along a marked-out 20-metre course six days a week for 12 weeks. There was a large number of drop-outs in this study, which highlights the need for support and perhaps group involvement. As the authors noted in this study, many patients felt uncomfortable performing their exercises in their local area.

In contrast, a home-based programme of resistance and endurance training in patients about to undergo lung volume reduction surgery (LVRS) showed good, clinically and statistically significant improvements in walking distance and health-related quality of life (Debigare et al. 1999). More impressively, there was minimal supervision with only two hours of face-to-face instruction provided, the remaining supervision being by telephone contact. However, the authors recommend caution in extrapolation of these data to the larger population of patients with COPD, since this group was highly motivated in preparation for surgery.

Home rehabilitation may be an effective strategy for patients who are unable to attend an outpatient or community programme, but drawbacks include a lack of group support, problems with monitoring, time and cost implications, and smaller overall gains (Garrod 1998). One advantage that appears to be associated with home programmes is that of adherence. One study comparing home care to hospital care suggests that improvements are sustained for longer if training occurs at home (Strijbos et al. 1996).

Community rehabilitation programmes provided in groups may be more effective (Cambach et al. 1999); however, we must ensure that any special needs are first met, that programmes are adequate and instructors are able to support the patient with cognitive-behavioural approaches that can enhance training. Strong links with community therapists and private leisure centres are essential to foster innovations. It is likely that for some patients initial attendance at a local leisure centre will be too overwhelming and that the hospital environment may provide reassurance for severely disabled patients (Garrod 1998). It is important to remember that COPD is a heterogeneous disease: what is right for one patient may be wrong for another.

Thus, the assessment process of pulmonary rehabilitation is the essential first step. From this we can identify individual patient needs and concerns, preferences and previous experiences. The assessment serves many purposes, not least evaluation of the benefits of the programme. It also serves to enable the patient to monitor and play a part in the management of his condition, and it allows an opportunity for the multidisciplinary team to specifically target appropriate action from within the relevant personnel. At present in the United Kingdom, assessment is often performed by one member, and an individualization of patient requirements is not always fully addressed. A thorough, multidisciplinary assessment will enhance practice: involving the community team ensures that new behaviours learnt in the outpatient programme can be practised in the home environment. If weakness plays a significant role in activity limitation, referral to a local gym may be appropriate; if anxiety is a particular problem, the patient may need greater psychosocial input and/or referral to a psychologist.

If all this sounds like pie in the sky, we need to think again. If our approach is collaborative, the numbers of available personnel will be increased, our management will be more effective and duplication of services can be minimized. And, most importantly, the patients will receive the seamless 'continuum of services' that they deserve.

The following chapters of this book will present issues of relevance to all health care professionals involved in the provision of pulmonary rehabilitation. There will be chapters devoted to the assessment of training, to the delivery of a training programme, the assessment of health-related quality of life and the part that rehabilitation plays in quality of life. There are also chapters devoted to the role of the occupational therapist, the role of the respiratory nurse, nutritional management, medical management and the psychological implication and management of respiratory disease. Much of this book will be reassuring for many of the readers: much good work is being done in pulmonary rehabilitation; however, there are things we can work on and improve, enabling an evaluative multidisciplinary approach that will enhance practice. It is hoped that this book will enable members of the multidisciplinary team to more clearly define their role and state their commitment to achieving and maintaining the individual's maximum level of independence and functioning in the community.

References

Agusti AG, Noguera A, Sauleda J et al. (2003) Systemic effects of chronic obstructive pulmonary disease. European Respiratory Journal 21(2): 347–360.

Anonymous (1995) Clinical competency guidelines for pulmonary rehabilitation professionals: American Association of Cardiovascular and Pulmonary Rehabilitation Position Statement. Journal of Cardiopulmonary Rehabilitation 15(3): 173–178.

Anonymous ACCP/AACVPR (1997) Pulmonary Rehabilitation Guidelines Panel. 'Pulmonary rehabilitation: joint ACCP/AACVPR evidence-based guidelines.' Chest 112(5): 1363–1396.

Barach AL (1974) Chronic obstructive lung disease: postural relief of dyspnea. Archives of Physical Medicine and Rehabilitation 55(11): 494–504.

Bernard S, Leblanc P, Whittom F et al. (1998) Peripheral muscle weakness in patients with chronic obstructive pulmonary disease. American Journal of Respiratory and Critical Care Medicine 158(2): 629–634.

British Thoracic Society (BTS) (2001) Statement on Pulmonary Rehabilitation. Thorax 56: 827–834.

British Thoracic Society (BTS) website: http: //www.brit-thoracic.org.uk

Busch AJ, McClements JD (1988) Effects of a supervised home exercise programme on patients with severe chronic obstructive pulmonary disease. Physical Therapy 68(4): 469–474.

Cambach W, Wagenaar RC, Koelman TW et al. (1999) The long-term effects of pulmonary rehabilitation in patients with asthma and chronic obstructive pulmonary disease: a research synthesis. Archives of Physical Medicine and Rehabilitation 80(1): 103–111.

Cole TM, Fishman AP (1994) Workshop on pulmonary rehabilitation research: a commentary. American Journal of Physical Medicine and Rehabilitation 73(2): 132-133.

Debigare R, Maltais F, Whittom F et al. (1999) Feasibility and efficacy of home exercise training before lung volume reduction. Journal of Cardiopulmonary Rehabilitation 19(4): 235–241.

Garrod R (1998) Pulmonary rehabilitation: the pros and cons of rehabilitation at home. Physiotherapy 84(12): 603–607.

Garrod R, Bestall JC, Paul EA et al. (2000) Development and validation of a standardized measure of activity of daily living in patients with severe COPD: the London Chest Activity of Daily Living Scale (LCADL). Respiratory Management 94(6): 589–596.

Gosselink R, Troosters T, Decramer M (1996) Peripheral muscle weakness contributes to exercise limitation in COPD. American Journal of Respiratory and Critical Care Medicine 153(3): 976–980.

Griffiths TL, Phillips CJ, Davies S et al. (2001) Cost effectiveness of an outpatient multidisciplinary pulmonary rehabilitation programme. Thorax 56(10): 779–784.

Hamilton AL, Killian KJ, Summers E et al. (1995) Muscle strength, symptom intensity, and exercise capacity in patients with cardiorespiratory disorders. American Journal of Respiratory and Critical Care Medicine 152(6 part 1): 2021–2031.

Hernandez MT, Rubio TM, Ruiz FO et al. (2000) Results of a home-based training programme for patients with COPD. Chest 118(1): 106–114.

Hodgkin JE, Farrell MJ, Gibson SR et al. (1982) American Thoracic Society. Medical Section of the American Lung Association. Pulmonary rehabilitation. American Review of Respiratory Disease 124(5): 663–666.

Lacasse Y, Guyatt GH, Goldstein RS (1997) The components of a respiratory rehabilitation program: a systematic overview. Chest 111(4): 1077–1088.

Make BJ (1986) Pulmonary rehabilitation: myth or reality? Clinical Chest Medicine 7(4): 519–540.

Maltais F, Jobin J, Sullivan MJ et al. (1998) Metabolic and hemodynamic responses of lower limb during exercise in patients with COPD. Journal of Applied Physiology 84(5): 1573–1580.

Maltais F, Leblanc P, Simard C et al. (1996) Skeletal muscle adaptation to endurance training in patients with chronic obstructive pulmonary disease. American Journal of Respiratory and Critical Care Medicine 154(2 part 1): 442–447.

McGavin CR, Gupta SP, Lloyd EL et al. (1977) Physical rehabilitation for the chronic bronchitic: results of a controlled trial of exercises in the home. Thorax 32(3): 307–311.

Morey S (2000) American Thoracic Society updates statement on pulmonary rehabilitation. American Family Physician 61(5): 1550–1552.

Morgan MDL, Calverley PMA, Clark CJ et al. (2001) BTS Statement: Pulmonary Rehabilitation. Thorax 56(11): 827–834.

O'Donnell DE, McGuire M, Samis L et al. (1998a) General exercise training improves ventilatory and peripheral muscle strength and endurance in chronic airflow limitation. American Journal of Respiratory and Critical Care Medicine 157(5 part 1): 1489–1497.

O'Donnell DE, Lam M, Webb KA (1998b) Measurement of symptoms, lung hyperinflation, and endurance during exercise in chronic obstructive pulmonary disease. American Journal of Respiratory and Critical Care Medicine 158(5 part 1): 1557–1565.

Petty TL (1968) Training in respiratory care. American Review of Respiratory Disease 98(6): 1060–1061.

Schols AM, Slangen J, Volovics L et al. (1998) Weight loss is a reversible factor in the prognosis of chronic obstructive pulmonary disease. American Journal of Respiratory and Critical Care Medicine 157(6 part 1): 1791–1797.

Sharp JT, Drutz WS, Moisan T et al. (1980) Postural relief of dyspnea in severe chronic obstructive pulmonary disease. American Review of Respiratory Disease 122(2): 201–211.

Strijbos JH, Postma DS, van Altena R et al. (1996) A comparison between an outpatient hospital-based pulmonary rehabilitation programme and a home-care pulmonary rehabilitation programme in patients with COPD: a follow-up of 18 months. Chest 109(2): 366–372.

Toevs CD, Kaplan RM, Atkins CJ (1984) The costs and effects of behavioral programs in chronic obstructive pulmonary disease. Medical Care 22(12): 1088–1100.

Wedzicha JA, Bestall JC, Garrod R et al. (1998) Randomized controlled trial of pulmonary rehabilitation in severe chronic obstructive pulmonary disease patients, stratified with the MRC dyspnoea scale. European Respiratory Journal 12(2): 363–369.

Whittom F, Jobin J, Simard PM et al. (1998) Histochemical and morphological characteristics of the vastus lateralis muscle in patients with chronic obstructive pulmonary disease. Medicine and Science in Sports and Exercise 30(10): 1467–1474.

World Health Organization (2001) International Classification of Functioning. http: //www.who.int/dsa/justpub/ICFFlierA.pdf

Chapter 2
Selection of patients: who benefits?

M. DECRAMER, R. GOSSELINK, T. TROOSTERS

Introduction

Chronic obstructive pulmonary disease (COPD) is a slowly progressive disorder characterized by irreversible airflow obstruction and enhanced annual decline in lung function (Siafakas et al. 1995). At present, only smoking cessation has been shown to affect the decline in lung function (Anthonisen et al. 1994), while inhaled corticosteroids cause a small increment in lung function and quality of life, without, however, affecting this annual decline (Burge et al. 2000, Pauwels et al. 1999). One of the most important findings in the Inhaled Steroids in Obstructive Lung Disease in Europe (ISOLDE) study was the demonstration of an accelerated decline in health status in COPD patients with moderate to severe airflow obstruction (Burge et al. 2000). This decline in health status was confirmed in other studies.

Pulmonary rehabilitation programmes have become increasingly popular in the treatment of COPD during the past few years, although they have been available for several decades. Indeed, the review by Lertzman and Cherniack (1976) already had 184 references, clearly demonstrating the interest in the area more than 20 years ago. The treatment is, therefore, not new. What is new is that what can be expected from pulmonary rehabilitation programmes is now much clearer. This has been clarified in several randomized well-designed studies conducted during the past ten years, clearly demonstrating that pulmonary rehabilitation improves health status and functional exercise capacity in COPD patients. In addition, a multitude of observations has been made indicating that exercise capacity is poorly related to airflow obstruction in COPD patients, and that associated phenomena such as deconditioning and muscle weakness are important in generating symptoms in these patients. In the light of these observations, more clarity may also emerge on how candidates for a pulmonary rehabilitation programme should be selected. This will be discussed in the present chapter. Although several studies have examined this question in the past decade, the criteria that may be used in clinical practice remain very general and qualitative rather than quantitative.

The present chapter will essentially focus, therefore, on two questions:

1. What benefits can be expected from a rehabilitation programme?
2. How should candidates for pulmonary rehabilitation be selected?

Which benefits can be expected from a pulmonary rehabilitation programme?

Several well-designed studies published during the past ten years have answered a number of important questions related to what can be expected from pulmonary rehabilitation programmes. It is now abundantly clear that pulmonary rehabilitation reduces symptoms (O'Donnell et al. 1993), improves exercise tolerance (Toshima, et al. 1990, Goldstein et al. 1994, Griffiths et al. 2000, Troosters et al. 2000, Ries et al. 1995) and improves quality of life in COPD patients (Goldstein et al. 1994, Griffiths et al. 2000, Troosters et al. 2000, Ries et al. 1995). The latter effects were reviewed in a meta-analysis by Lacasse et al. (1996). In this meta-analysis, quality of life was measured in 12 out of 14 trials considered. However, only two validated instruments were used: the transitional dyspnoea index and the chronic respiratory disease questionnaire, CRDQ. The CRDQ was used in four trials (Goldstein et al. 1994, Simpson et al. 1992, Wijkstra et al. 1994, Güell et al. 2000). As a whole, quality of life improved in all four of its dimensions: dyspnoea, fatigue, emotional function and mastery. The average increase observed exceeded the minimal clinically important difference for all of these dimensions. Moreover, for the dimensions dyspnoea and mastery the minimal effect also exceeded the minimal clinically important difference (MCID) set at 0.5 points on a Likert-type score comprising seven points. Examples of effects of rehabilitation on six-minute walking distance (6-MWD) and health status we recently obtained (Troosters et al. 2000) are shown in Figures 2.1 and 2.2.

Six important trials were also published but were not included in meta-analysis by Lacasse et al. (1996) (Toshima et al. 1990, Griffiths et al. 2000, Troosters et al. 2000, Ries et al. 1995, Wedzicha et al. 1998, Criner et al. 1999). The first of these trials (Ries et al. 1995) did not show an improvement in quality of life, but it demonstrated an improvement in the symptoms of dyspnoea and fatigue. The absence of an effect on quality of life, however, is likely to be due to the fact that a generic quality of life instrument, the quality of well-being scale, was used. Indeed, this instrument is less sensitive than the disease-specific instruments. Two of these trials used the St George's Respiratory Questionnaire (SGRQ) in combination with the CRDQ and found an effect of rehabilitation that in one study might have been less pronounced in patients with severe dyspnoea (Wedzicha et al. 1998). The last trial used the Sickness Impact Profile (SIP)

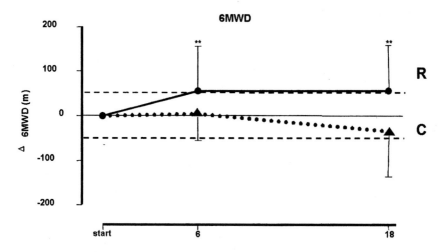

Figure 2.1 Effects of a six-month outpatient rehabilitation programme on 6-MWD. The rehabilitation group (R) is represented by the solid line and the control group (C) by the dotted line. The effect clearly exceeds the minimal clinically important difference of about 55 metres, shown by the dashed line. From Troosters et al. (2000). ** p < 0.01.

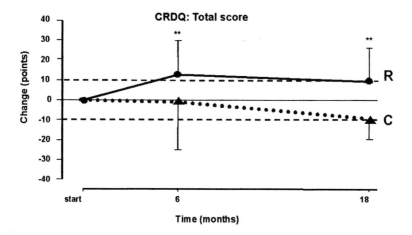

Figure 2.2 Effects of a six-month outpatient rehabilitation programme on health status measured with the CRDQ. The rehabilitation group (R) is represented by the solid line and the control group (C) by the dotted line. The effect clearly exceeds the minimal clinically important difference shown by the dashed line. The effects on the total score are shown; similar effects were obtained in the four subdomains. From Troosters et al. (2000).** p < 0.01.

and found that eight weeks' rehabilitation as well as LVRS (Criner et al. 1999) improved quality of life. Three months of additional rehabilitation did not further improve quality of life after an eight-week programme, while LVRS did. It is noteworthy that the SIP is also a generic instrument that probably lacks sensitivity. Moreover, it should be noted in this trial that the effects of rehabilitation on functional exercise capacity were exceedingly small, averaging about 16 meters. This is considerably less than the effect of rehabilitation programmes on functional exercise capacity commonly observed and averaging about 55 meters (Lacasse et al. 1996). This probably signals that either the patients had already undergone rehabilitation before the eight-week programme, thus resulting in better physical condition before the programme, or that the programme was too short and not intensive enough. This observation is of considerable importance as similar effects were observed in the NETT-trial (Make et al. 2000).

It is now also well established that improvements in exercise capacity and quality of life obtained after rehabilitation are poorly related (Troosters et al. 2000, Reardon et al. 1993). In a recent study, we demonstrated reasonable relationships between the improvements in quality of life measured with the CRDQ and the improvements in muscle force following rehabilitation (Troosters et al. 2000). This might signal that muscle force is one of the key variables in pulmonary rehabilitation, allowing the establishment of links that hitherto were unexplained. Moreover, it is not necessary to improve exercise capacity to observe improvements in quality of life. Indeed, Simpson et al. (1992) demonstrated that weightlifting exercise, training the peripheral muscles without affecting exercise capacity, clearly improved all four dimensions of the CRDQ. Similarly, we recently showed that aerobic exercise training and peripheral muscle strength training improved health status, as measured by the CRDQ, to a similar extent in COPD patients with peripheral muscle weakness (Spruit et al. 2002).

At present, pulmonary rehabilitation has not been shown to improve survival in COPD patients, although at least two studies have shown tendencies for improved survival after pulmonary rehabilitation (Ries et al. 1995, De Paepe et al. 2000). As it appears no longer ethical to randomize patients to a control group, it will be difficult to examine this matter further in methodologically robust trials. A meta-analysis of the three available trials may contribute to further elucidation of this issue. In addition, two recent studies (Griffiths et al. 2000, Troosters et al. 2000) demonstrated reductions in the number of hospital admissions and reductions in the number of hospital days. The study by Griffiths et al. (2000) demonstrated a concomitant increase in the number of visits to the general practitioner, pointing to an enhanced use of primary-care facilities. This increase may signal that the patients use health care more appropriately after the programme as they would judge their own condition better. These findings are all the more relevant since COPD patients are known to be high consumers of health care resources (Strauss 1986, Grasso et al. 1998). Finally, a recent cost–utility analysis demonstrated that the incremental cost–utility ratio was negative, indicating that the rehabilitation programme was paid for by the reduction of the utilization of health care resources caused by the programme. A high likelihood of generating Quality Adjusted Life Years (QALYS – the cost associated with an additional year's survival at optimum quality of life) at a negative or relatively low cost was found (Griffiths et al. 2001.)

How should we select candidates for pulmonary rehabilitation?

If pulmonary rehabilitation beneficially affects outcome variables in COPD patients, should we then admit all COPD patients into these programmes or should we select patients? If so, how should we select patients for admission into pulmonary rehabilitation programmes? At present, there are clearly fewer data on how to select candidates than on the overall beneficial effects of pulmonary rehabilitation. In addition, it appears to be quite an attractive idea to direct rehabilitation to those activities of daily living that pose most problems to a particular patient. This 'selective' training, however, has, to the best of our knowledge, never really been critically examined. In addition, it is not clear that such specific training would be more effective than a general training programme. Although it appears intuitively likely that this specific training would be the way forward in COPD, we shall in the present chapter address only general rehabilitation programmes.

A number of prerequisites before admission are generally claimed. It is expected that medical therapy is optimized and that the patient stops smoking or at least enrols in a smoking-cessation programme, since smoking cessation is at present the only treatment known to affect the evolution of COPD (Anthonisen et al. 1994). There is, however, at present no evidence that the beneficial effects of training programmes would be smaller in smokers. For further selection, a number of studies trying to predict the outcome after pulmonary rehabilitation may be useful to consider.

A study by ZuWallack et al. (1991) was one of the first studies trying to predict the improvement in 12-minute walking distance (12-MWD) occurring after pulmonary rehabilitation in 50 severe COPD patients. This improvement was related to the initial 12-MWD, the peak oxygen consumption, the peak oxygen pulse, and the ventilatory reserve at peak exercise. Hence, patients with a lower exercise capacity at the onset who do not exhibit ventilatory limitation would be the better candidates. In multiple regression analysis, only the initial 12-MWD and FEV_1 had predictive power regarding the response of the 12-MWD. It should be stressed that in this study the relationship between improvement in 12-MWD and baseline 12-MWD poses a statistical problem and that the regression coefficient obtained in the present study is likely to be overestimated. In subsequent studies, the usefulness of FEV_1 as a selection criterion has been clearly debated.

Indeed, Maltais et al. (1997) demonstrated that training responses were similar in COPD patients with an FEV_1 above and below 40 per cent of predicted FEV_1. The effects on ventilation and heart rate at a VO_2 max corresponding to the pretraining maximum, peak oxygen consumption and maximal workload were all similar. Only the reduction in lactate at the pretraining maximum was slightly different between the two groups. In addition, the study showed that workload and training time clearly increased in the first four weeks of training in these patients, such that after four weeks decent training loads (60 per cent max) and times (20 minutes) were obtained, which were perfectly capable of bringing about physiological training effects in the heart and muscles. Training effects were even found in patients with hypercapnia (Foster et al. 1988). A study by Casaburi et al. (1997) also showed that training effects were readily obtained in patients with severe COPD who were not capable of raising their lactate levels during exercise much above 2 mmol/L. A similar observation was made by Punzal et al. (1991), who demonstrated that patients who did not reach their anaerobic threshold during training improved as much as those who did. This is an important insight of the past years and has significant consequences for the applicability of pulmonary rehabilitation as a whole. Indeed, since patients with severe airflow obstruction also appear to improve substantially after a training programme, a rehabilitation programme is an important treatment option in end-stage COPD either alone or in preparation for lung transplantation or LVRS. In our institution, patients are considered for these surgical procedures only when they successfully complete a rehabilitation programme. The effects obtained in these patients challenge the old idea that beneficial effects of exercise training were expected only in those patients who were capable of increasing their lactic acid levels substantially during exercise. At present, there is no longer any basis for this contention.

In a recent study, we analysed the predictors of training effects in a group of 82 COPD patients following a six-month outpatient rehabilitation programme (Troosters et al. 2001). Response was defined as a 15 per cent increase in maximum workload and/or a 25 per cent increase in 6-MWD. In general, 32 (65 per cent) out of the 49 patients responded to the treatment. Responders were characterized by lower handgrip force, maximal inspiratory pressure (PImax), 6-MWD, maximal workload, heart rate and ventilation at peak exercise. The differences between responders and non-responders are summarized in Table 2.1.

The pretraining ratio handgrip force, ventilatory reserve determined by VEmax/MVV (ventilation/maximal voluntary ventilation), 6-MWD, maximal workrate (Wmax) and PImax, were related to the subsequent response. In discriminant analysis only the ratio VEmax/MVV, peripheral muscle force and PImax contributed significantly to the distinction between responders and non-responders. The non-responder group showed more ventilatory limitation and had peripheral and respiratory muscle function closer to normal before starting rehabilitation. It should be emphasized, however, that only 32 per cent of the variance was explained by the discriminant model. This means that it is difficult to predict the response to a training programme from the baseline functional characteristics. As a

Table 2.1 Differences in functional characteristics between 32 responders and 17 non-responders to a rehabilitation programme

	Responders	Non-responders
n	32	17
FEV$_1$ (% pred)	36 ± 15	39 ± 14
TL,CO (% pred)	49 ± 26	50 ± 27
QF (% pred)	76 ± 28	79 ± 19
HF (% pred)	82 ± 25	100 ± 17**
PImax (% pred)	64 ± 19	80 ± 24*
6-MWD (% pred)	49 ± 17	63 ± 20**
Load (Watt)	59 ± 30	91 ± 33**
HRmax (% pred)	81 ± 13	90 ± 12**
VE/MVV (%)	90 ± 23	112 ± 34**
CRDQtot (AU)	74 ± 18	79 ± 14

TL,CO = transfer capacity, QF = quadriceps force, HF = handgrip force, PImax = maximal inspiratory pressure, HRmax = maximal heart rate, VE/MVV = ratio of maximal exercise ventilation to maximal voluntary ventilation, CRDQtot = total score on the CRDQ. * $p < 0.01$

consequence, it is important to apply a trial treatment to observe whether patients improve with the treatment. Hence, in the present state of the art, it is not possible to use functional variables at the onset of the programme as a selection criterion.

A number of other factors that may be related to response have been studied in recent years. Comprehensive outpatient and in-patient pulmonary rehabilitation was as beneficial in older patients with COPD as in younger patients (Couser et al. 1995). Longer-term rehabilitation was shown to be more effective than shorter-term in men, but not in women (Foy et al. 2001). Benefits might be smaller in patients with more severe dyspnoea than in patients with less severe dyspnoea, although the programme delivered in these two groups was different (Wedzicha et al. 1998). Patients who did not adhere to the programme were shown to be more socially isolated, lack COPD-related social support, still smoking, and less compliant with other health care activities such as the use of inhaled corticosteroids (Young et al. 1999). Improvements were shown to be less in patients with the greatest tendency to use wishful thinking as a coping strategy (Büchi et al. 1997).

In general, the following intuitive and empirical rules may be proposed in the knowledge that the studies presently available do not really offer a sound basis to distinguish responders from non-responders accurately. As a whole, we would select patients who have symptomatic respiratory disease resulting in reduced health status and decreased functional status. The patients need to be motivated to attend a pulmonary rehabilitation programme. Although no clear data are available supporting this requirement, and patient motivation may change in the course of the programme, it appears obviously important from clinical practice. Finally, they should not have co-morbidity that might interfere with the rehabilitation process (e.g. uncontrolled rheumatoid arthritis) or that places the patient at an excessive risk during exercise training (e.g. unstable ischemic cardiovascular disease) (ZuWallack 1998, Morgan 1999). As outlined above, patients with any level of airflow obstruction are all candidates for rehabilitation programmes. This also means that patients in preparation for volume reduction surgery or transplantation are good candidates for rehabilitation.

Future research may be directed towards a better understanding of the response to rehabilitation. It was clearly shown that in some COPD patients signs of systemic inflammation are present (di Francia et al. 1994, Schols et al. 1996). In frail, elderly COPD patients, expression of tumour necrosing factor-alpha (TNF-α) in the vastus lateralis was enhanced compared to young controls, and diminished with strength training (Greiwe et al. 2001). It may be hypothesized that the patients with the greater systemic and local expression of TNF-α or other cytokines, such as IL-6 or IL-8, may not respond as well to rehabilitation as those with the lowest expression. This hypothesis is intriguing but requires further prospective validation.

An empirical clinical rule may be the following (Decramer et al. 1998): patients with moderate airflow obstruction with an FEV_1 between 40 per cent and 60 per cent predicted, with severe complaints of dyspnoea, impaired health status and clear peripheral muscle weakness constitute good candidates. A programme in such a patient would consist primarily of endurance training, peripheral muscle training, psychosocial support and dietary measures if they were either clearly underweight or overweight. The need for education, psychosocial support, ergotherapy or chest physiotherapy may be real, but is at present not clearly supported by available data.

From the programmes in preparation of lung transplantation (Fournier and Derenne 1995) or volume reduction surgery, it appears that patients with more severe airflow obstruction, with an FEV_1 between 20 and 40 per cent predicted, may also be good candidates for pulmonary rehabilitation, if presenting with severe complaints of dyspnoea, reduced health status, and severe peripheral muscle weakness. The programme in these patients should be directed towards peripheral muscle training, interval training (which may be a valid alternative to endurance training) and nutritional support (Coppoolse et al. 1999).

Conclusion

Although it has clearly been shown that pulmonary rehabilitation results in beneficial effects in COPD patients, it remains relatively difficult to develop sound grounds for the proper selection of candidates for these programmes. Muscle weakness, poor functional exercise capacity, and significant ventilatory reserve at peak exercise appear to be predictors of response. They, however, explain only a relatively small fraction of the variance in the response. The practical attitude appears to be to identify candidates for programmes on the basis of simple and empirical clinical rules. This means that patients with significantly reduced quality of life, and functional status of any degree of airflow obstruction, who are sufficiently motivated and who do not present contraindications are suitable candidates. Future research may help to identify better the patients who will respond on the basis of pre-rehabilitation data.

Acknowledgements

The studies cited in the present chapter were supported by the 'Fonds voor Wetenschappelijk Onderzoek-Vlaanderen' grants # G.0175.99 and G.0237.01 and by the Research Foundation of the Katholieke Universiteit Leuven, grant # OT 98/27. They were further supported by AstraZeneca pharmaceuticals.

References

Anthonisen NR, Connett JE, Kiley JP et al. (1994) Effects of smoking intervention and the use of anticholinergic bronchodilator on the rate of decline of FEV-1. The lung health study. Journal of Medical Association 272(19): 1497–1505.

Büchi S, Villiger B, Sensky T et al. (1997) Psychosocial predictors of long-term success of inpatient pulmonary rehabilitation of patients with COPD. European Respiratory Journal 10(6): 1272–1277.

Burge PS, Calverley PMA, Jones PW et al. (2000) Randomized, double blind, placebo controlled study of fluticasone propionate in patients with moderate to severe chronic obstructive pulmonary disease: the ISOLDE trial. British Medical Journal 320(7245): 1297–1303.

Casaburi R, Porszasz J, Burns MB et al. (1997) Physiologic benefits of exercise training in rehabilitation of patients with severe chronic obstructive pulmonary disease. American Journal of Respiratory and Critical Care Medicine 155(5): 1541–1551.

Coppoolse R, Schols AMWJ, Baarends EM et al. (1999) Interval versus continuous training in patients with severe COPD: a randomized clinical trial. European Respiratory Journal 14(2): 258–263.

Couser JI, Guthmann R, Hamadeh MA et al. (1995) Pulmonary rehabilitation improves exercise capacity in older elderly patients with COPD. Chest 107(3): 730–734.

Criner GA, Cordova FC, Furukawa S et al. (1999) Prospective randomised trial comparing bilateral lung volume reduction surgery to pulmonary rehabilitation in severe chronic obstructive pulmonary disease. American Journal of Respiratory and Critical Care Medicine 160(6): 2018–2027.

Decramer M, Donner CF, Schois AMWJ (1998) Rehabilitation. In: Postma DS, Siafakas NM (eds.) Management of chronic obstructive pulmonary disease. European Respiratory Monograph 3: 215–234.

De Paepe K, Troosters T, Gosselink R et al. (2000) Determinants of survival in patients with COPD (abstract). European Respiratory Journal 16 (Supplement 13): 31S.

Di Francia M, Barbier D, Mege JL et al. (1994) Tumor necrosis factor-alpha levels and weight loss in chronic obstructive pulmonary disease. American Journal of Respiratory and Critical Care Medicine 150(5 Part 1): 1453–1455.

Foster S, Lopez D, Thomas III HM (1988) Pulmonary rehabilitation in COPD patients with elevated PCO_2. American Review of Respiratory Disease 138(6): 1519–1523.

Fournier M, Derenne JPH (1995) Exercise performance in lung transplant candidates and recipients. European Respiratory Journal 5: 38–41.

Foy CG, Rejeski J, Berry MJ et al. (2001) Gender moderates the effects of exercise therapy on health-related quality of life among COPD patients. Chest 119(1): 70–76.

Goldstein RS, Gort EH, Stubbing D et al. (1994) Randomised controlled trial of respiratory rehabilitation. Lancet 344(8934): 1394–1397.

Grasso ME, Weller WE, Shaffer TJ et al. (1998) Capitation, managed care and chronic obstructive pulmonary disease. American Journal of Respiratory and Critical Care Medicine 158(1): 133–138.

Greiwe JF, Cheng B, Rubin DC et al. (2001) Resistance exercise decreases skeletal muscle tumor necrosis factor α in frail elderly humans. The Federation of American Societies for Experimental Biology Journal 15(2): 475–482.

Griffiths TL, Burr ML, Campbell IA et al. (2000) Results at 1 year of outpatient multidisciplinary pulmonary rehabilitation: a randomised controlled trial. Lancet 355(9201): 362–368.

Griffiths TL, Phillips CJ, Davies S et al. (2001) Cost effectiveness of an outpatient multidisciplinary pulmonary rehabilitation programme. Thorax 56(10): 779–784.

Güell R, Morante F, Sangenis M et al. (2000) Effects of respiratory rehabilitation on the effort capacity and on health-related quality of life of patients with chronic obstructive pulmonary disease. Chest 117: 976–983.

Lacasse Y, Wong E, Guyatt GH et al. (1996) Meta-analysis of respiratory rehabilitation in chronic obstructive pulmonary disease. Lancet 348(9035): 1115–1119.

Lertzman R, Cherniack RS (1976) Rehabilitation of patients with chronic obstructive pulmonary disease. State of the art. American Review of Respiratory Disease 114(6): 1145–1163.

Make B, Tolliver R, Christensen P et al. (2000) Pulmonary rehabilitation improves exercise capacity and dyspnea in the National Emphysema Treatment Trial (NETT). American Journal of Respiratory and Critical Care Medicine 161: A254.

Maltais F, Leblanc P, Jobin J et al. (1997) Intensity of training and physiologic adaptation in patients with chronic obstructive pulmonary disease. American Journal of Respiratory and Critical Care Medicine 155(2): 555–561.

Morgan MDL (1999) The prediction of benefit from pulmonary rehabilitation: setting, training intensity and the effect of selection by disability. Thorax 54(Supplement 2): S3–S7.

O'Donnell DE, Webb KA, McGuire MA (1993) Older patients with COPD. Benefits of exercise training. Geriatrics 48(1): 59–66.

Pauwels RA, Löfdahl CG, Laitinen LA et al. (1999) Long-term treatment with inhaled budesonide in persons with mild COPD who continue smoking. European Respiratory Society Study on Chronic Obstructive Pulmonary Disease. New England Journal of Medicine 340(25): 1948–1953.

Punzal PA, Ries AL, Kaplan RM et al. (1991) Maximum intensity exercise training in patients with chronic obstructive pulmonary disease. Chest 100(3): 618–623.

Reardon J, Patel K, ZuWallack RL (1993) Improvement of quality of life is unrelated to improvement in exercise endurance after outpatient pulmonary rehabilitation. Journal of Cardiopulmonary Rehabilitation 13: 51–54.

Ries AL, Kaplan RM, Limberg TM et al. (1995) Effects of pulmonary rehabilitation on physiologic and psychosocial outcomes in patients with chronic obstructive pulmonary disease. Annals of Internal Medicine 122(11): 823–832.

Schols AMWJ, Buurman WA, Staal-van den Brekel AJ et al. (1996) Evidence for a relation between metabolic derangements and increased levels of inflammatory mediators in a subgroup of patients with chronic obstructive pulmonary disease. Thorax 51(8): 819–824.

Siafakas NM, Vermeire P, Pride NB et al. (1995) Optimal assessment and management of COPD. European Respiratory Journal 8(8): 1398–1420.

Simpson K, Killian K, McCartney N et al. (1992) Randomised controlled trial of weightlifting exercise in patients with chronic airflow limitation. Thorax 47(2): 70–75.

Spruit MA, Gosselink R, Troosters T et al. (2002) Resistance versus endurance training in patients with COPD and peripheral muscle weakness. European Respiratory Journal 19(6): 1072–1078.

Strauss MJ (1986) Cost and outcome of care for patients with chronic obstructive lung disease. Medical Care 24(10): 915–924.

Toshima MT, Kaplan RM, Ries AL (1990) Experimental evaluation of rehabilitation in chronic obstructive pulmonary disease: short-term effects on exercise endurance and health status. Health Psychology 93(3): 237–252.

Troosters T, Gosselink R, Decramer M (2000) Short and long-term effects of outpatient rehabilitation in chronic obstructive pulmonary disease: a randomised controlled trial. American Journal of Medicine 109(3): 207–212.

Troosters T, Gosselink R, Decramer M (2001) Exercise training in COPD: how to distinguish responders from nonresponders. Journal of Cardiopulmonary Rehabilitation 21(1): 10–17.

Wedzicha JA, Bestall JC, Garrod R et al. (1998) Randomized controlled trial of pulmonary rehabilitation in severe chronic obstructive pulmonary disease patients, stratified with the MRC dyspnoea scale. European Respiratory Journal 12(2): 363–369.

Wijkstra PJ, van Altena R, Kraan J et al. (1994) Quality of life in patients with chronic obstructive pulmonary disease after rehabilitation at home. European Respiratory Journal 7(2): 269–273.

Young P, Dewse M, Fergusson W et al. (1999) Respiratory rehabilitation in chronic obstructive pulmonary disease: predictors of nonadherence. European Respiratory Journal 13(4): 855–859.

ZuWallack RL (1998) Selection criteria and outcome assessment in pulmonary rehabilitation. Monaldi Archives Chest Diseases 53(4): 429–437.

ZuWallack RL, Patel K, Reardon JZ et al. (1991) Predictors of improvement in the 12-minute walking distance following a six-week outpatient pulmonary rehabilitation programme. Chest 99(4): 805–808.

Chapter 3
Health-related quality of life and pulmonary rehabilitation

J. BESTALL

Introduction

Health-related quality of life (HRQoL) questionnaires aim to measure a range of concepts concerning the person, their health and their perceived well-being. The development of HRQoL measures has been important for health care professionals and patients, since these measures focus on patient-centred issues. HRQoL measures may complement objective clinical markers of health, and in some cases replace them as the more appropriate measure. This has proved particularly true for the field of pulmonary rehabilitation, where it is well known that objective measures, such as lung-function tests, do not accurately reflect observed changes in health. The main reason for this is that pulmonary rehabilitation programmes can improve symptoms, fitness and well-being but are unable to influence the overall anatomical and physiological problems experienced by patients. The subsequent use of field and laboratory exercise tests and symptom scores revealed that patients with chronic obstructive pulmonary disease (COPD) could benefit from pulmonary rehabilitation in terms of improvements in walking distance and perception of breathlessness (Make 1986). However, the measurement of symptoms alone did not represent the totality of the patient's experience of their condition.

Definition of HRQoL

The definition of HRQoL has been the subject of debate since it may encompass more than just health-related issues. A simple definition is 'The gap between that which is desired and that which is achievable' (Calman 1984). This provides us with an idea of the kind of concept that HRQoL questionnaires try to address. However, it is not clear enough for us to know exactly what the producers of such questionnaires are trying to measure. To understand this, we need to consider the use of the term 'quality of life' and why it is useful to refer to 'health-related quality of life' or 'health status'.

Why measure HRQoL

One of the major criticisms of HRQoL is based on the relationship between measures of pulmonary function and health status. These relationships are at best weak; however, Curtis et al. (1994) suggest that if 'hard' physiological measures accurately reflected the entirety of a person's health status, there would be no need for HRQoL measures. The fact that these relationships are weak but that these measures are detecting something suggests that in complex chronic illness there is more occurring than just physiological changes. Variability in function, mood state and physiological symptoms cannot be summed up using only one measure. Jones (1995) reports that there was no single measure of lung function that could summarize the disturbances that may cause breathlessness in patients with COPD. This has indicated the need for the use of a number of assessments covering the basic problems associated with COPD.

HRQoL or health status?

Health services researchers are primarily interested in measuring the perceptions of health experienced by a large number of patients. They require measures that assess a person's health perception in a standardized manner and which can be used for comparisons between groups of patients. The main reason for the requirement of standardized instruments is to compare populations of patients. This has led to a difference in terminology, where some HRQoL measures are referred to as 'health status assessments'. Health status may be thought of as a more accurate term since quality of life may encompass more than just one's health-related issues. Health status has thus been further defined as, 'The quantification of the impact of disease on daily life and perceived well-being in a formal and standardized manner' (Jones 1991).

For the purposes of this chapter, we shall refer to 'HRQoL', but this may encompass quality of life and health status. These terms should all be used when searching health and social databases for such measures.

Individualization or standardization?

Quality of life may be said to encompass the whole of a person's life, including not only their health but also social and family life plus religious or spiritual beliefs. It does not strictly assess health perception. The list of items that are important to any particular individual are unique and complex (Allison et al. 1997). This could be perceived as a problem since the measurement of uniquely individual characteristics can be relevant only for that individual. The only way in which to measure an individual's quality of life is to determine which features of life are important to that person and for them to weight each of these features according to importance in their life. This process has been utilized by McGee et al. (1991), who developed the Schedule for Evaluation of Individual Quality of Life (SEIHRQoL). However, although the questionnaire was effective for assessing the individual, it was limited in that it was extremely subjective, comparable only within individuals, and was very time-consuming. This type of measure is therefore not useful for assessing population health in research. Further, its use in clinical practice may be limited due to the administration time involved. This study is a good example of a generic questionnaire designed for individuals. However, at the other end of the spectrum are questionnaires designed for measuring the health of whole populations of patients. Such questionnaires may be used to determine the average response of a sample of patients to a particular intervention. A good example of such a questionnaire is the St George's Respiratory Questionnaire (SGRQ) (Jones et al. 1991). This is a disease-specific questionnaire originally developed for use in asthma and COPD. It was designed to be used in large populations of patients and has shown good results in a number of settings (Jones 1991, Jones 1995, Spencer et al. 2001).

Generic questionnaires versus disease-specific questionnaires

HRQoL was initially measured with generic health measures such as the Sickness Impact Profile (SIP) (Bergner et al. 1981), the quality of well-being scale (QWS) (Kaplan 1984) and the Medical Outcomes Study Short Form-36 (MOS SF-36) (Ware and Sherbourne 1992). Generic measures of HRQoL may be administered to patients with different diagnoses, e.g. heart failure, asthma or arthritis. Such measures allow comparisons between groups of patients but do not assess a single problem in depth. However, the MOS SF-36 has shown good results following a pulmonary rehabilitation programme (Griffiths et al. 2000). In contrast to this, a number of disease-specific questionnaires have been developed. Disease-specific measures have been designed for use in one particular problem or a group of related problems. The disease-specific questionnaires that have been designed for patients with respiratory illnesses are:

1. The chronic respiratory disease questionnaire (CRDQ) (Guyatt et al. 1987)
2. The St George's Respiratory Questionnaire (SGRQ) (Jones et al. 1991)
3. The Breathing Problems Questionnaire (BPQ) (Hyland et al. 1994)
4. The Quality of Life in Respiratory Illness Questionnaire (HRQoLRIQ) (Maille et al. 1997).

These measures assess a number of health-related issues including symptoms, psychosocial status, daily activity and self-efficacy. Further, they have contributed to an increased understanding of the patient's perception of their illness. The use of these measures has also enabled us to assess patient-centred issues in a formal and standardized manner.

Questionnaire design and development

The development of any questionnaire should be based on sound psychometric principles. It is beyond the scope of this chapter to describe these principles in detail, and only a basic summary is provided. However, the reader is directed to other sources (especially Streiner and Norman 1995, and Bowling 2001) for more information about the process of questionnaire development and the types of outcomes that are currently available. In general terms, one would expect that a questionnaire should have published data concerning the reliability, the validity and the sensitivity of the new measure. The assessment of reliability, validity and sensitivity are complex processes. However, it is necessary to understand such concepts in order to critically evaluate quality of life measures.

Reliability

A good quality of life questionnaire should be reliable (also referred to as *repeatability*). A questionnaire may be said to be reliable when it demonstrates consistent results over short time periods with the same respondents and administrators. There are numerous methods for testing reliability, including test–retest reliability, intra-rater and inter-rater agreement and tests of internal consistency such as split-half, item–item correlations and item–total correlations.

Test–retest reliability

The simplest method of estimating reliability requires the administration of the same test to the same group of people on two different occasions. The reliability is estimated simply by working out the correlation between the two sets of scores. This method is known as the test–retest method. The rationale behind this method is that, since each test is administered twice and every test is parallel with itself, differences between scores on the test and on the retest should be due solely to measurement error. Unfortunately, this argument is often inappropriate for psychological or health attributes since it is often impossible to consider the second administration of a test as a parallel measure to the first. Thus it may be inaccurate to treat test–retest correlation as a measure of reliability and instead to use only a split-half reliability where the test data are split into two and the two halves are correlated with one another, e.g. Cronbach's alpha (Cronbach 1951).

Internal consistency

Internal consistency measures, such as Cronbach's alpha (Cronbach 1951), assess the homogeneity of the items included in the questionnaire and indicate whether the questions are from the same conceptual domain. A low co-efficient alpha (<0.50) indicates that the questions are not from the same conceptual domain (Bowling 2001). Where a questionnaire is concerned with more than one domain of health, it may be necessary to include more than one concept and therefore Cronbach's alpha is less appropriate, and factor analysis should be employed to determine the components of the questionnaire.

Inter-observer agreement

This refers to the differences in measurement achieved by different administrators of the measure. This may be measured using the Kappa statistic (Cohen 1960), which assesses the proportion of responses that are agreed by two observers, taking into account that some of the agreements may occur by chance. Inter-observer differences will be examined both within the same professional groups (e.g. community nurses with the same patient) and between different professional groups (e.g. the GP and community nurse assessing the same patient).

One further aspect of reliability is the ability of the measure to differentiate between patients. A quality of life measure, if administered to an adequate sample of patients, should display good discriminatory properties. For example, it should demonstrate that there are some patients with poor quality of life scores, some with medium scores and some with relatively good scores in terms of the impact of their condition on their daily life and well-being.

Validity

There are many types of validity testing that occur at different stages of questionnaire development and use.

Face and content validity

A good quality of life questionnaire should accurately reflect the issues relating to the condition (in this case COPD) in which it may be used. A questionnaire is said to demonstrate good face validity if it appears to be measuring the construct of interest (face validity is a simple assessment of whether the questionnaire looks right). Content validity refers to the extent to which the questionnaire accurately represents specific aspects of a condition or illness (e.g. physical aspects such as symptoms, or activities and psychosocial aspects such as mastery of illness, or the effect on the patient's life).

Concurrent validity

In an ideal world, once the questionnaire had been developed, there would be a gold standard that could be used to assess how well the new questionnaire would perform. The comparison of a new measure to a gold standard is known as 'criterion validity'. However, as there usually is no gold standard, it is common to choose a number of measures that reflect the different aspects of the patient's condition. These may be other questionnaires or subsets of questionnaire and may include measures such as lung function. This is known as measuring the *concurrent validity* of a questionnaire. The results demonstrate how the new measure is similar to and/or different from to other measures.

Predictive validity

Once the questionnaire has been developed, it may be used in practice to predict prognosis or survival. In these instances, the questionnaire is used as part of a research study using cohorts of patients to determine performance.

Sensitivity

The sensitivity of a measure can be determined by administering the questionnaire to a group of patients before and after an intervention, usually within a clinical trial setting. The subsequent change in score will reveal whether a questionnaire can adequately measure small but clinically significant changes over time in longitudinal trials. If a questionnaire has been found to be sensitive to change, it is important that investigators define the minimal clinical significant difference since this may not always be the same as statistical significance for any particular intervention.

Measuring quality of life

It is usual to measure quality of life over two time points, e.g. before a pulmonary rehabilitation programme and after the end of a programme. This allows one to determine the change in score or the size of effect on HRQoL. This change may be analysed by applying statistical tests and estimating confidence intervals or p-values to calculate the amount of statistical precision of this change. However, what is a meaningful change for a quality-of-life measure? A change in FEV_1 of a few litres is easy to understand, but it is much more difficult to imagine what a meaningful change in quality of life would be, since there is no specific unit of HRQoL. This has led to the development of the minimum clinical important difference (MCID). The MCID is calculated by asking patients, clinicians or other raters to subjectively rate whether they think a patient or they themselves have benefited from an intervention. These ratings are then compared to the actual changes in the scores of the patient to determine the change scores of those that have improved. This process has been carried out for both the CRDQ and the SGRQ. The MCID for the SGRQ is a change of four points, for the CRDQ it is an average change of 0.5 per domain. A meta-analysis of pulmonary rehabilitation by Lacasse et al. examined HRQoL in a number of trials. They found that all the domains of the CRDQ improved by the MCID and that the specific components – dyspnoea and mastery – improved by more than the MCID (Lacasse et al. 1996). This was illustrated by a diagram that showed that the 95% confidence interval for these components did not cross the MCID, providing evidence that pulmonary rehabilitation provides patients with significant benefit. Further discussion of MCIDs may be found in the literature (Redelmeier 1996, Wright 1996).

Types of instrument

There are three main types of health status measure. First, there are utility scales, which try to measure the impact of different health states. These measures rate each illness on a scale between perfect health and death. Although suitable for economic analysis, since death is included in the scale, these measures are less precise in terms of sensitivity to change (Jones 1995). Second, there are generic measures that are used for comparison across different disease populations. Generic measures were originally designed to define the health of populations and not to measure the efficacy of particular interventions. These measures have been used for the latter and have proved to be useful for assessing patients with mild COPD but have not proved as effective for patients with more severe disease (Jones 1995). Such instruments may be limited since they attempt to include many populations within one instrument, which means that the scoring bands for each group are quite narrow. Also, it is difficult to judge the impact of one disease compared with another, considering the multi-factorial influences of each illness. The work with generic measures identified a need for more disease-specific instruments. This led to the development of disease-specific questionnaires for patients with asthma and COPD. These questionnaires are similar to generic measures, though their scope is widened since the whole scale relates to only one disease population. Table 3.1 shows a range of measures used to assess HRQoL.

Quality of life and pulmonary rehabilitation

There have been a number of studies in COPD that have included a quality of life assessment. The range of disease severity studied is from 30 to 70 per cent predicted FEV_1 (McSweeney et al. 1989, Prigatano et al. 1984,

Table 3.1 HRQoL measures used in the assessment of patients with COPD

	Type	Method of use	Time (mins)	Domains
SIP (Bergner et al. 1981)	generic	self-rated	15	sleep and rest, emotion, self-care, housework, mobility, family and friends, walking, stairs, feelings, communication
QWS (Kaplan et al. 1984)	generic	interview (training)	15–20	mobility, physical activity, social activity, worst symptom
Nottingham Health Profile (Hunt et al. 1981)	generic	self-rated	15	part 1: physical, pain, mobility, sleep, energy, social isolation, emotion part 2: work, home, social, interests, holidays
MOS SF-36 Health Survey (Ware and Sherbourne 1992)	generic	self-rated	10–15	physical functioning, role function, bodily pain, general health, vitality, social functioning, role-emotional, mental health
CRDQ (Guyatt et al. 1987)	disease-specific	interview (training)	20–25	dyspnoea, emotional function, fatigue, mastery
SGRQ (Jones et al. 1991)	disease-specific	self-rated	10–15	symptoms, activity, impact, total
BPQ (Hyland et al. 1994)	disease-specific	self-rated	10–15	walking, bending/reaching, effect of temperature, household effects of smells/fumes/cold, sleeping, medicine, dysphoric states, (constructs: health knowledge, health appraisal)

Ketelaars et al. 1996). Patients with COPD have widely variable levels of disease severity in terms of FEV_1 and respiratory disability and tend to show the same patterns with quality of life. The largest disturbances in HRQoL as described by McSweeney et al. (1989) were domains of emotional disturbance (mainly depression), recreational activities, home management, sleep and rest.

Investigators have found varying results with measures of HRQoL of patients with COPD who had attended a rehabilitation programme (Wijkstra et al. 1994, Ries et al. 1995). Ries et al. found no differences between their exercise and control groups for HRQoL assessed by the QWS. However, this was probably due to the fact that this instrument was not disease specific and was less sensitive to change in patients with severe COPD. In contrast, Wijkstra et al. (1994) found that the patients who received an exercise intervention had good improvements in their health status assessed by the CRDQ. A meta-analysis of pulmonary rehabilitation noted that each study appeared to use a different quality of life assessment, which made the comparison of these studies difficult (Lacasse et al. 1996). This study highlighted the fact that pulmonary rehabilitation tended to have the largest significant effect on two aspects of quality of life – namely dyspnoea and mastery as measured by the CRDQ.

There have been four studies that have measured more than one of the most commonly used HRQoL measures including both generic and disease-specific measures (Wedzicha et al. 1998, Harper et al. 1997, Singh et al. 2001, Griffiths et al. 2000). The study by Wedzicha et al. (1998) reports that the CRDQ produced better results than the SGRQ after an eight-week programme of pulmonary rehabilitation. However, the study was stratified using the Medical Research Council dyspnoea scale to account for the differing levels of respiratory disability, thus dividing the study into two halves; furthermore, this study was not primarily powered to detect changes in HRQoL measured by the SGRQ. A further study by Harper et al. (1997) assessed the use of generic measures: the MOS SF-36, the EUROQoL, and the disease-specific measures: the CRDQ and SGRQ. They assessed the validity of each and found them all to be reliable measures. However, they noted that the generic measures were more useful for picking up other problems (perhaps in terms of co-morbidity) than the disease-specific questionnaires. Griffiths et al. (2000) measured both the SGRQ and the CRDQ after a six-week pulmonary rehabilitation programme plus follow-up in 200 patients. They reported that both measures showed significant improvements after a pulmonary rehabilitation programme. Finally, Singh et al. (2001) carried out a study where they compared the three most commonly used disease-specific questionnaires (CRDQ, SGRQ and BPQ) and the two most common generic measures (a global quality of life scale and an activity checklist). They reported that, overall, the CRDQ was the most sensitive to change following a pulmonary rehabilitation programme. However, they report results from non-randomized studies, and the effects of bias should be considered in relation to their results.

Table 3.2 provides the reader with some examples of randomized studies of pulmonary rehabilitation. These studies vary in a number of ways in terms of the settings in which the rehabilitation programme was carried out, the types of training provided, and the duration of the programme. Most studies compared rehabilitation to standard therapy, with only two studies comparing rehabilitation to an education programme (Ries et al. 1995, Wedzicha et al. 1998). Overall, the most commonly used measure was the CRDQ, which generally showed that patients with COPD would

Table 3.2 Quality of life and pulmonary rehabilitation

Author	Setting	Duration	Compared to	HRQoL measure	Results
Busch and McClements 1988	home	18 weeks	standard therapy	CRDQ (dyspnoea only)	No difference Small sample and attrition
Simpson et al. 1992	outpatient	8 weeks	standard therapy	CRDQ	Improvements in two components of CRQ
Goldstein et al. 1994	in-patient	8 weeks	standard therapy	CRDQ	Improvements in CRQ
Wijkstra et al. 1994	home	3 months plus follow-up for 18 months	standard therapy	CRDQ	Improvements in CRQ after 3 months and up to 18 months (small numbers and intensive programme)
Ries 1995	outpatient	8 weeks	education	QWB scale	No improvement in this generic measure
Guell 2000	outpatient	3 months	standard therapy	CRDQ	Improvements after programme maintained up to 24 months
Wedzicha et al. 1998	outpatient and home	8 weeks + one year follow up	education	CRDQ, SGRQ	Improvement in CRQ in outpatient group after programme and at six months
Ringbaek et al. 2000	outpatient	8 weeks	standard therapy	CRDQ	No improvement (low numbers of patients)
Griffiths et al. 2000	outpatient		standard therapy	CRDQ, SGRQ, MOS SF-36	Improvement in all measures. Good sample
Troosters et al. 2000	outpatient	6 months +18 months	standard therapy	CRQ	Improved CRQ at 6 months not maintained at 18 months
Finnerty et al. 2001	outpatient	6 weeks	standard therapy	SGRQ	Improved after 6 weeks and maintained at 24 weeks

have adequate-to-good changes in HRQoL scores immediately after the programme and with extended training periods. Although few studies have utilized the SGRQ, it too has generally shown good results post-rehabilitation where the studies are powered to assess change in SGRQ.

Research tool or clinical practice tool?

There has been a lot of debate about the types of outcome that ought to be measured, both in clinical trials and in the working practice of clinicians. In real terms, the requirements of research and the require-ments of working practice are different both in terms of the processes each may require and in terms of the overall outcome. One of the key questions asked by practising therapists is whether they could use research questionnaires in practice. Answering this is not easy, since there are a number of factors to consider. In a lot of cases, questionnaires designed for use in a research setting will be too long and complex for a shorter assessment. However, it is useful to check whether the question-naire has been validated in different settings or may have been modified to be used in a clinical setting. For example, the BPQ has been modified for use in clinical practice with the shortened version having been shown to be as useful as the original (Hyland et al. 1998). A very simple and quick assessment for respiratory illness is the Airways Questionnaire 20 (AQ20) (Barley et al. 1998). This is a 20-item instrument that takes only a few minutes to complete. It has been validated for use in asthma (Barley et al. 1998) and COPD (Hajiro et al. 1999) and takes only two or three minutes to complete. A review by Jones (2001) further addresses this problem. He uses evidence from quality of life research to develop a set of key components that can be used in clinical history taking to quick-ly assess whether the patient feels they have benefited from their treatment.

When to use a quality-of-life measure in clinical practice

It is most important that the questionnaire be able to provide you with the type of data that you require, and provide answers to the questions that you want to assess. As in all cases the outcome should be appropri-ate. Higginson and Carr (2001) have described when HRQoL could be used in clinical practice. They describe six potential clinical uses of HRQoL measures; these are:

- to prioritize problems
- to facilitate communication
- to screen for potential problems

- to identify preferences
- to monitor changes or responses to treatment
- to train new staff.

HRQoL measures should be used to ensure that treatment plans and evaluations are patient centred rather than disease centred. It must be remembered that HRQoL is not the only type of assessment available. Other appropriate measures are activity of daily living or functional status questionnaires, measures of disability, or psychological assessments. The choice of measure should be relevant to the type of information that you require.

References

Allison PJ, Locker D, Feine JS (1997) Quality of life: a dynamic construct. Social Science and Medicine 45(2): 221–30.

Barley EA, Quirk FHJPW (1998) Asthma health status measurement in clinical practice: validity of a new short and simple instrument. Respiratory Medicine 92(10): 1207–14.

Bergner M, Bobbitt RA, Carter WB et al. (1981) The Sickness Impact Profile: development and final revision of a health status measure. Medical Care 19(8): 787–805.

Bowling A (2001) Measuring Health: A review of quality of life measurement scales. Buckingham: Open University Press.

Busch AJ, McClements JD (1988) Effects of a supervised home exercise program on patients with severe chronic obstructive pulmonary disease. Physical Therapy 68(4): 469–74.

Calman KC (1984) Quality of life in cancer patients – a hypothesis. Journal of Medical Ethics 10(3): 124–127.

Cohen J (1960) A co-efficient of agreement for nominal scales. Educational and Psychological Measurement 20: 37–46.

Chronbach LJ (1951) Co-efficient alpha and the internal structure of tests. Psychometrika 16: 297–334.

Curtis JR, Deyo RA, Hudson LD (1994) Pulmonary rehabilitation in chronic respiratory insufficiency. 7. Health-related quality of life among patients with chronic obstructive pulmonary disease. Thorax 49(2): 162–170.

EuroQol (1990) A new facility for the measurement of health-related quality of life. The EuroQol Group. Health Policy 16(3): 199–208.

Finnerty JP, Keeping I, Bullough I et al. (2001) The effectiveness of outpatient pulmonary rehabilitation in chronic lung disease: a randomized controlled trial. Chest 119(6): 1705–10.

Goldstein RS, Gort EH, Stubbing D et al. (1994) Randomised controlled trial of respiratory rehabilitation. Lancet 344(8934): 1394–1397.

Griffiths TL, Burr ML, Campbell IA et al. (2000) Results at 1 year of outpatient multidisciplinary pulmonary rehabilitation: a randomised controlled trial. Lancet 355(9201): 362–368.

Guell R, Casan P, Belda J et al. (2000) Long-term effects of outpatient rehabilitation of COPD: a randomized trial. Chest 117(4): 976–983.

Guyatt GH, Berman LB, Townsend M et al. (1987) A measure of quality of life for clinical trials in chronic lung disease. Thorax 42(10): 773–778.

Hajiro T, Nishimura K, Jones PW et al. (1999) Novel, short, and simple questionnaire to measure health-related quality of life in patients with chronic obstructive pulmonary disease. American Journal of Respiratory and Critical Care Medicine 159(6): 1874–1878.

Harper R, Brazier JE, Waterhouse JC et al. (1997) Comparison of outcome measures for patients with chronic obstructive pulmonary disease (COPD) in an outpatient setting. Thorax 52(10): 879–887

Higginson IJ, Carr AJ (2001) Using quality of life measures in the clinical setting. British Medical Journal 322(7297): 1297–1300.

Hunt SM, McKenna SP, McEwen J et al. (1981) The Nottingham Health Profile: subjective health status and medical consultations. Social Science and Medicine[A] 15(3 Part 1): 221–229.

Hyland ME, Bott J, Singh S et al. (1994) Domains, constructs and the development of the breathing problems questionnaire. Quality of Life Research 3(4): 245–256.

Hyland ME, Singh SJ, Sodergren SC et al. (1998) Development of a shortened version of the Breathing Problems Questionnaire suitable for use in a pulmonary rehabilitation clinic: a purpose-specific, disease-specific questionnaire. Quality of Life Research 7(3): 227–233.

Jones PW (1991) Quality of life measurement for patients with disease of the airways. Thorax 46: 682.

Jones PW (1995) Issues concerning health related quality of life in Chronic Obstructive Pulmonary Disease. Chest 107(Supplement 5): 187S–193S.

Jones PW (2001) Health status measurement in COPD. Thorax 56(11): 880–887.

Jones PW, Quirk FH, Baveystock CM (1991) The St Georges Respiratory Questionnaire (SGRQ). Respiratory Medicine 85(Supplement B): 25–31.

Kaplan RM, Atkins CJ, Timms R (1984) Validity of a quality of well-being scale as an outcome measure in COPD. Journal of Chronic Diseases 37(2): 85–95.

Ketelaars CAJ, Shlosser MAG, Mostert R et al. (1996) Determinants of health-related quality of life in patients with COPD. Thorax 51(1): 39–43.

Lacasse Y, Wong E, Guyatt GH et al. (1996) Meta-analysis of respiratory rehabilitation in chronic obstructive pulmonary disease. Lancet 348(9035): 1115–1119.

Maille AR, Koning CJ, Zwinderman AH et al. (1997) The development of the Quality-of-Life for Respiratory Illness Questionnaire (QOL-RIQ): a disease-specific quality-of-life questionnaire for patients with mild to moderate chronic non-specific lung disease. Respiratory Medicine 91(5): 297–309.

Make BJ (1986) Pulmonary rehabilitation: myth or reality? Clinical Chest Medicine 7(4): 519–540.

McGee HM, O'Boyle CA, Hickey A et al. (1991) Assessing the quality of life of the individual: the SEIQOL with a healthy and a gastroenterology unit population. Psychological Medicine 21(3): 749–759.

McSweeney AJ, Grant I, Heaton RK et al. (1989) Life quality of patients with COPD. Kango Gijutsu 35(5): 572–582 (Japanese).

Prigatano GP, Wright EC, Levin D (1984) Quality of life and its predictors in patients with mild hypoxaemia and COPD. Archives of Internal Medicine 144(8): 1613–1619.

Redelmeier DA, Guyatt GH, Goldstein RS (1996) Assessing the minimal important difference: a comparison of two techniques. Journal of Clinical Epidemiology 49(11): 1223–1224.

Ries AL, Kaplan RM, Limberg TM et al. (1995) Effects of pulmonary rehabilitation on physiologic and psychosocial outcomes in patients with chronic obstructive pulmonary disease. Annals of Internal Medicine 122(11): 823–832.

Ringbaek TJ, Broendum E, Hemmingsen L et al. (2000) Rehabilitation of patients with chronic obstructive pulmonary disease. Exercise twice a week is not sufficient! Respiratory Medicine 94(2): 150–154.

Simpson K, Killian K, McCartney N et al. (1992) Randomised controlled trial of weightlifting exercise in patients with chronic airflow limitation. Thorax 47(2): 70–75.

Singh SJ, Sodergren SC, Hyland ME et al. (2001) A comparison of three disease-specific and two generic health-status measures to evaluate the outcome of pulmonary rehabilitation in COPD. Respiratory Medicine 95(1): 71–77.

Spencer S, Calverley PMA, Burge PS et al. (2001) Health status deterioration in patients with COPD. American Journal of Respiratory and Critical Care Medicine 163(1): 122–128.

Streiner DL, Norman GR (1995) Health Measurement Scales: a practical guide to their development and use. Oxford: Oxford University Press.

Troosters T, Gosselink R, Decramer M (2000) Short- and long-term effects of outpatient rehabilitation in patients with chronic obstructive pulmonary disease: a randomized trial. The American Journal of Medicine 109(3): 207–212.

Ware JE, Sherbourne CD (1992) The MOS 36-Item Short-Form Health Survey (SF-36). Medical Care 30(6): 473–483.

Wedzicha JA, Bestall JC, Garrod R et al. (1998) Randomized controlled trial of pulmonary rehabilitation in severe chronic obstructive pulmonary disease patients, stratified with the MRC dyspnoea scale. European Respiratory Journal 12(2): 363–369.

Wijkstra PJ, van Altena R, Kraan J et al. (1994) Quality of life in patients with COPD improves after rehabilitation at home. European Respiratory Journal 7(2): 269–273.

Wijkstra PJ, Ten Vergert EM, van Altena R et al. (1995) Long-term benefits of rehabilitation at home on quality of life and exercise tolerance in patients with chronic obstructive pulmonary disease. Thorax 50(8): 824–828.

Wright JG (1996) The minimal important difference: who's to say what is important? Journal of Clinical Epidemiology 49(11): 1221–1222.

Chapter 4
Exercise prescription and training

C. CLARK, L. COCHRANE, S. CONROY

Introduction

There have been several very helpful guidelines published recently on pulmonary rehabilitation both in the United Kingdom (BTS 2001) and North America (ATS 1999) and also an excellent guideline focusing on exercise management of patients across a wide spectrum of diseases entitled *Exercise Management for Persons with Chronic Diseases and Disabilities* (American College of Sports Medicine 2002). These are combined with our own experience in this field to provide the following review of the requirements for exercise prescription in patients with chronic lung disease. The general principles and the process of exercise prescription are generic, i.e. common to persons with chronic diseases and disabilities of various types and adapted from programmes used in training otherwise healthy but sedentary normal subjects. The principle is that there should first be definition of the individual person's problems with particular reference to participation in physical activity and, second, a realistic plan should be designed to optimize the individual's exercise participation in order that specific identifiable goals can then be achieved. The choice of goals must therefore be identified at the outset. These can broadly be defined as:

1. *improvement of cardiorespiratory fitness* as defined by established physiological criteria (such as improved VO_2max, increased stroke volume, and increased efficiency of peripheral oxygen extraction)
2. *improved exercise tolerance* empirically, i.e. without necessarily achieving significant changes in the above physiological criteria
3. *simple conditioning designed to retain and improve mobility*, focusing on a programme of utilization of muscles, plus allied joints, tendons and ligaments, of the kind achieved by simple callisthenics.

In addition to exercise training, comprehensive, pulmonary rehabilitation programmes need to address three other major components:

education, psychosocial/behavioural intervention and outcome assessment. These interventions are generally provided by a multidisciplinary team, which varies in size but increasingly includes physicians, nurses, physiotherapists, occupational therapists, nutritionists, psychologists and social workers. Exercise training is the most essential component required to improve the tolerance of activities of daily living (ATS 1999), but the pervasive nature of the disability seen across the spectrum of disease severity means that a comprehensive approach is required to optimize therapeutic options.

Exercise training

Exercise training is the foundation of pulmonary rehabilitation. Although exercise has to date not resulted in measurable improvements in underlying respiratory impairment (airways obstruction on lung-function testing), its positive effects on dyspnoea during exercise, for example, underscore the importance of physical deconditioning as a co-morbid factor heightening disability in advancing lung disease. Physical training may have a central desensitizing effect on the sensation of breathlessness. Rhythmic, repetitive exercise can produce improvements in electroencephalographic synchronicity (Fernal and Daniels 1984) and can increase endorphin levels without reducing ventilatory chemosensitivity. (Mahler et al. 1989). An analogy can be drawn between this and the type II effects of drugs, such as chlorpromazine, that reduce breathlessness by a central effect that is independent of changes in ventilation (Stark 1988).

(Whole-body) exercise training

The general principles of exercise physiology as applied to normal individuals (American College of Sports Medicine 1986) state that, where the required outcome is improved fitness, the extent of benefit obtained is dependent on training intensity, frequency, duration, programme length, specificity of exercises undertaken and reversibility, i.e. the effects of interruption or cessation of training on the changes achieved.

In healthy subjects, aerobic or fitness training is usually targeted at 60 to 90 per cent of the predicted maximal heart rate or 50 to 80 per cent of the maximal oxygen uptake. This level is sustained for 20 to 45 minutes, and repeated three to five times a week. Training at this intensity, which is usually well above the anaerobic threshold, increases maximal exercise performance, causes physiological adaptations that improve oxygen extraction in peripheral muscles and enhance cardiac function (specifically stroke volume) in healthy subjects (Holloszy and Coyle 1984). Until recently, patients with advanced lung disease such as chronic obstructive pulmonary disease (COPD) have been considered to have a ventilatory limitation that would preclude the intensity of aerobic training levels necessary for such beneficial physiologic adaptations (Belman and Kendregan 1982).

The training intensity chosen in early studies was often well below the level of workrate required. However, later studies have demonstrated that anaerobic metabolism and an early onset of lactic acidosis can be observed in exercise training of patients with COPD (Casaburi et al. 1991, Maltais et al. 1996) with greater improvements in maximal and submaximal exercise responses obtained after exercise training at high (60 per cent of maximal workrate above the anaerobic threshold) compared to low (30 per cent of maximal workrate) exercise levels (Casaburi et al. 1991). Increases in oxidative enzymes in the peripheral muscles indicative of physiological adaptation to training have been found after strenuous (Maltais et al. 1996) but not low-intensity training (Belman and Kendregan 1982), and reductions seen in levels of ventilation and the blood lactate produced at identical submaximal workrates following high-intensity exercise training suggest that adaptations of aerobic metabolism are attainable in many patients with COPD (Casaburi et al. 1991), provided that they can tolerate the level of programme intensity. Training respiratory patients at 60 to 75 per cent of predicted maximal workrate (calculated indirectly from training heart rate expressed as a percentage of maximal heart rate, which in turn usually approximates to the simple formula: max. heart rate = 210 − age (American College of Sports Medicine 1986), results in substantial increases in maximal exercise capacity and in some cases reductions in ventilation and lactate levels at identical exercise workrates (Maltais et al. 1996, Maltais et al. 1997). Additionally, changes in heart rate at a standardized submaximal workrate can be used to study cardiac adaptations after exercise training in patients with COPD (Casaburi et al. 1991, Maltais et al. 1996, Casaburi et al. 1997).

The relationship between heart rate and workrate, however, varies widely among subjects (Katch et al. 1978) and may be affected by cardiac and lung disease or their therapy (Wasserman et al. 1994). Despite these limitations, heart rate measured at a given percentage of peak workrate is a reasonable approximate parameter to set training intensity targets and thereafter to monitor progress in the individual patient. Most pulmonary rehabilitation programmes emphasize high-intensity steady-state endurance training as the paradigm, utilizing periods of sustained exercise for about 20 to 30 minutes, two to five times a week. An overall programme duration of six to 12 weeks is recommended (Casaburi et al. 1997, Wijkstra et al. 1996, Cambach et al. 1997, Maltais et al. 1997), and the longer-duration programmes in our experience tend to encourage compliance with subsequent exercise self-management by the patient in the community on completion, perhaps because patient attitudes and knowledge have received reinforcement due to the extended time of exposure to the programme.

Virtually all the physiological gains can be expected to be achieved in the first six weeks and, therefore, constraints on the availability of places on the programme may be the deciding factor influencing duration offered at various centres. While training at 60 per cent of the maximal workload for prolonged periods of time is possible for a proportion of patients with severe airways obstruction (Ries et al. 1995, Casaburi et al. 1991), many *cannot* tolerate training at this intensity (Maltais et al. 1996, Maltais et al. 1997). In these patients, alternative approaches have to be considered, such as interval training, consisting of two to three minutes of high-intensity (60–80 per cent maximal exercise capacity) training alternating with equal or longer periods of rest. In healthy subjects, interval training elicits training effects similar to endurance training (Poole and Gaesser 1985, Debusk et al. 1990), but, to date, its role in patients with lung disease is unclear (Schols et al. 1996) including information regarding tolerability and therefore applicability across the spectrum of disease severity.

Another alternative is to *adjust the goal desired* for these patients towards simply *improving tolerability of exercise at higher levels than previously* without expecting to achieve the physiological adaptations specifically associated with improved cardiorespiratory fitness. This approach can be expected to aid patients in performing daily activities at the very least, and in some cases might be a useful springboard from which to progress to a higher-intensity programme subsequently. In this approach, the patient would work at the highest tolerable level of steady-state exercise determined by the trainer empirically during introductory sessions, with repeated measures of heart rate being used to reproduce that level of exercise performance during subsequent training sessions. Dyspnoea ratings, for example the Borg Breathlessness Scale or visual analogue scale (VAS), during maximal graded exercise testing may reliably predict specific exercise intensities during training (Horowitz et al. 1996), making symptom-targeted exercise training a possible alternative to heart rate-targeted training (O'Donnell et al. 1995, Punzal et al. 1991). In this case, the highest tolerable exercise intensity would again be determined empirically and the patient would learn to adjust intensity according to their own responses during exercise sessions.

Training specificity

Training specificity refers to the observation that benefit is usually gained only in those activities involving the muscle groups that are specifically trained. For instance, an increase in the six-minute walk distance (6-MWD) occurs with lower-extremity training but not with upper-extremity training (Lake et al. 1990). There is, however, some transfer effect to other activities, since cycle ergometer training improves walking distance (Cambach et al. 1997) and vice versa. Free walking is a natural way to ensure that commonly used muscle groups are engaged in the training process and, if gymnasium training is being used, attention must be given to a balance of upper-limb and lower-limb training. Endurance training of the upper extremities to improve arm function is potentially important since many activities of daily living involve use of the arms, and there is evidence of beneficial effects. Training using supported-arm exercises with ergometry, or unsupported-arm exercises by lifting free weights, dowels and stretching elastic bands can effectively improve arm endurance (Martinez et al. 1993). However, most pulmonary rehabilitation programmes emphasize endurance training of lower extremities, using singly or in combination stationary cycle exercise, treadmill walking or ground-based walking. Not only is there a considerable increase in submaximal endurance time with lower-extremity training of COPD patients, there is also a dose-response effect: higher-intensity exercise (60–80 per cent of the maximum workrate) is more effective than lower-intensity exercise (30 per cent of the maximal workrate) (Casaburi et al. 1991). Studies of cycle ergometer training (Maltais et al. 1996, Vallet et al. 1997), treadmill walking (Goldstein et al. 1994, Ries et al. 1995, Poole et al. 1985), or combined walking and cycling (O'Donnell et al. 1995) have consistently shown improvements in maximal workrate and submaximal endurance time.

Multigym (individual muscle group) strength and endurance training

Since peripheral muscle weakness contributes to exercise limitation in patients with lung disease (Hamilton et al. 1995) and can even cause falls and injury in the elderly or infirm, strength plus endurance training of individual muscle groups, particularly those supporting the main limb girdles, is a rational component of exercise training during pulmonary rehabilitation. Two randomized controlled studies (Simpson et al. 1992, Clark et al. 2000) suggest this may be a beneficial constituent of exercise training. Both were trials involving exercise for respiratory patients consisting of weightlifting submaximal loads repetitively over a programme duration, typical of whole-body endurance programmes, in an attempt to induce greater strength and endurance of the muscle groups. These showed that the group which exercised with loads approximating 60 per cent of the one-repetition maximum had a much greater increase in peripheral muscle function than an untreated control group, but, perhaps even more importantly in terms of potential practical relevance, there was a concomitant increase in whole-body submaximal exercise endurance in both studies, and there was an improvement in quality of life (health status) measures in the study in which this was measured (Simpson et al. 1992).

The principle involved in multigym training of specific muscle groups is repetition of isotonic contractions, i.e. against a fixed weight, usually 60 to 80 per cent of the maximum weight tolerated by the patient in a single contraction during preliminary testing by the physiotherapist (Astrand and Rhodahl 2003, Brown et al. 1990). There is an analogy with whole-body training in which submaximal exercise is used to induce endurance benefits in the muscles, and it should be noted that the use of the term 'weight training' should not be taken to mean simply the traditional anabolic approach designed to increase muscle bulk in weight, for example in weightlifters. A set of ten repetitions of each exercise is performed three times with a rest period between sets. Two circuit sessions a week are undertaken in the physiotherapy department and provision of a small mobile weights system allows a third session at home. All patients complete a circuit of the same exercises but with their own individual prescription (an example is given in Table 4.1). The order of exercises is not critical but must be preceded by a five-minute conditioning period of stretching exercises designed to prevent muscle, tendon and ligament injuries. This type of training does not require heart rate monitoring as the objective is not central cardiovascular conditioning but rather improving strength and endurance of individual muscle groups. The key to a successful outcome lies in the suitability of initial prescription and then physiotherapist guidance, particularly regarding the speed of repetitions and the length of rest periods between the stations.

The individual's response in terms of breathlessness is of paramount importance to the physiotherapist. Each patient is taught to use the Borg Breathlessness Scale (BBS) to guide the intensity and number of repetitions plus rest times. Before commencing each new exercise, the breathlessness score should have reduced to acceptable levels (in the case of the BBS this should be less than 3), i.e. adequate recovery time is necessary to allow tolerance of the whole range of circuit exercises. An example programme is given in Table 4.2.

Low-intensity muscle group training

This represents a potentially important alternative programme for patients with severe disease. Some of this group of patients will be unable to participate in whole-body endurance training or perhaps in multigym weight training. The adjusted objective must be to reduce the effects of major skeletal muscle deconditioning and loss of function due to enforced inactivity and poor nutritional status. These patients often have difficulty with the most basic of tasks, such as rising from bed, dressing, moving from room to room and washing themselves. The programme is designed to gently restore locomotor function of individual joint muscles, ligaments and tendons by a series of careful stretching exercises plus gentle repetitions of muscle contraction and relaxation. By exercising each muscle group *in isolation* and unloaded, breathlessness is minimized as is the risk of musculoskeletal injury. The programme given in Table 4.2 improves individual muscle strength, endurance, and mobility (Clark et al. 1996). This contains a range of upper- and lower-limb movements including simple modifications such as wall press-ups and sitting stomach-muscle exercises to avoid undue breathlessness due to posture, i.e. lying flat. The main attraction of such a programme is that it can be performed at home once learned under careful supervision. One physiotherapy session a week should be allocated to instruction of up to ten patients, and four weekly teaching sessions should suffice for each patient followed by home self-management of a daily 20-minute session thereafter.

Table 4.1 Multigym exercises designed to improve skeletal muscle strength and endurance

These exercises do not need to be performed in a set order. They must, however, be preceded by a five-minute period of warm-up exercises prescribed by the physiotherapist. Weight ranges are given for each item of equipment.

1. **Supine bench press**: exercises the chest, front of shoulders and rear upper arm.
Position: the patient lies with shoulders below the handlebar and presses upwards until elbows locked then returns to resting position.
Repetitions: 10 continuously over approximately 20 seconds. The breathing pattern should coincide with repetitions, breathe out on exertion, rest between sessions until the BBS is less than 3. Weight range 12 to 74 kg with 2 kg increments to 22 kg and 4 kg increments thereafter.

2. **Power squats**: exercise the buttocks, thighs and back.
Position: the patient stands facing the weights, squats down beneath shoulder pads and grabs bar and pushes up until knees lock straight then carefully returns to resting position.
Repetitions: breathing pattern and rest periods as for 1. Weight range 20 to 90 kg with 5 kg increments.

3. **Calf raises**: exercise the ankle extensors.
Position: at same equipment as for 2, stand with shoulders beneath the pads and knees straight and locked. Lift heels raising weights until fully extended on tips of toes only.
Repetitions: as for exercise 1. Weight range 20 to 90 kg with 5 kg increments.

4. **Latissimus pull down**: exercises the large back muscles, upper chest and front upper arms.
Position: stand facing weights, grasp overhead bar and pull down to mid-chest. Return carefully to resting position.
Repetitions: as for exercise 1. Weight range 0 to 70 kg with 5 kg increments.

5. **Upright rowing**: exercises the shoulder muscles and elbow flexors.
Position: stand facing the low pulley, draw weight to thighs then lift handlebar from thighs to shoulder height returning carefully to thighs.
Repetitions: as for exercise 1. Weight range 5 to 65 kg with increments of 2.5 kg to 15 kg then 5 kg increments.

6. **Leg press**: exercises all lower-limb muscles in co-ordinated fashion.
Position: sitting with knees bent and feet on rotating foot plate, push till knees fully extended leading with heels, not toes, then carefully return to resting position.
Repetitions: as for exercise 1 but allow 30 seconds for each set. Weight range 32 to 208 kg with 11 kg increments.

7. **Leg extension**: exercises the quadriceps.
Position: sit with back to weights and feet hooked under lower pads. Extend at knees until fully locked and return carefully to resting position.
Repetitions: as for exercise 6. Weight range 7 to 61 kg with 3 kg increments.

8. **Leg curls**: exercises the hamstrings.
Position: lie flat on bench face down with heels under padded roller. Curl legs till heels are directly above knees then carefully return to resting position.
Repetitions: as for exercise 6. Weight range 7 to 61 kg with 3 kg increments.

Table 4.2 Circuit of conditioning exercises designed to improve patient's strength and mobility

1. **Shoulder shrugging**: Circling shoulder girdle forward, down, backwards and up. Keep timing constant allowing 2 full seconds per circle. Relaxation encouraged throughout. Continue for 30 seconds.
Repeat the exercise 3 times with short rest intervals between sets until BBS is less than 3.

2. **Full-arm circling**: One arm at a time, passing arm as near as possible to side of the head, circle arm in as large a circle as possible. (Allow 8–10 seconds per circle.)
Repeat for 40 seconds continuously. Repeat the exercise 3 times with short rest intervals. Repeat with other arm.

3. **Increasing arm circles**: Hold arm away from body at shoulder height. Circle arms, progressively increase the size of circle for a count of 6 circles in 10 seconds then decrease for a further count of 6.
Repeat for 40 seconds. Repeat with other arm.

4. **Abdominal exercise**: Sitting in a chair, tighten abdominal muscles, hold for a count of 4 and then release muscles over 4 seconds to starting position.
Repeat continuously for 30 seconds. Perform the procedure 3 times with short rest periods in between.

5. **Wall press-ups**: Stand with feet a full-arm length distance from wall, place hands on wall and bend at elbow until nose touches wall, push arms straight again. Allow 8 seconds approximately from start to finish.
Repeat continuously for 40 seconds to a total of 5 repetitions. Perform the procedure 3 times with short rest periods in between.

6. **Sit to stand**: Using a dining-room chair, sit, stand, sit allowing for 8–10 seconds from start to completion. Use arms to assist stand only if unable to stand unassisted.
Repeat continuously for 40 seconds to a total of 5 repetitions. Perform the procedure 3 times with short rest periods in between.

7. **Quadriceps exercise**: Sitting on a chair, straighten right knee, tense thigh muscle, hold for a count of 4, then relax gradually over a further 4 seconds to a total of 5 repetitions over 40 seconds.
Repeat the exercise 3 times with short rest periods in between. Repeat procedure with left leg.

8. **Calf exercises**: Holding on to back of chair, go up on toes, return to floor taking 8 to 10 seconds to complete the procedure.
Repeat continuously for 40 seconds.

9. **Calf alternates walking on the spot**: Stand with feet about a foot apart. Holding on to back of chair, allow left knee to bend, keeping toes on ground. Bend right knee, while straightening left knee and allow 4 seconds for complete procedure.
Repeat this bending/straightening of knees and alternate knees, i.e.: walking on spot keeping toes on ground continuously for 40 seconds to a total of 10 repetitions. Repeat the exercise 10 times with short rest periods in between.

10. **Step-ups**: Step up with right foot on to step then bring up left foot. Step down with right foot then with left foot. Breathe out during step-up phase. Allow 4

seconds for the complete procedure and repeat continuously for 40 seconds. *Repeat* the exercise 3 times with short rest periods in between.

Exercises may be progressed by increasing the number of repetitions, increasing the speed at which they are performed, or reducing the rest periods.

In a trial of a low-intensity leg and arm muscle conditioning compared to an untreated control group (Clark et al. 1996), the treatment group increased their whole-body exercise performance and possibly had physiological adaptation to exercise, manifested by a reduced ventilatory equivalent for oxygen and carbon dioxide. No changes in maximal exercise performance were present or expected but, again, submaximal exercise endurance increased significantly.

Respiratory muscle training

Inspiratory muscle function may be compromised in COPD, an impairment that may contribute to dyspnoea (Hamilton et al. 1995), exercise limitation (Killian and Jones 1988) and hypercapnia (Begin and Grassino 1991). Respiratory muscle strength is commonly estimated by measuring maximal inspiratory pressure (PImax) (Black and Hyatt 1969), although this is a highly effort-dependent test. Inspiratory muscle training is generally initiated at low intensities then gradually increased to achieve 60 to 70 per cent of PImax. The minimal load required to achieve a training effect is 30 per cent of the PImax (Kim et al. 1993). Two methods of inspiratory muscle training most commonly used are threshold loading and resistive loading. With threshold loading, the training load is independent of flow (Larson et al. 1988, Gosselink et al. 1996), requiring the build-up of negative pressure before flow occurs, and hence is inert in nature. Threshold and resistive training effects have not been adequately compared. Although inspiratory muscle training using adequate loads undoubtedly improves strength of the inspiratory muscles in patients with COPD (Dekhuijzen et al. 1991, Harver et al. 1989), it remains unclear whether this results in a decrease in symptoms, disability or handicap. There is some evidence that improvement in inspiratory muscle strength in COPD is accompanied by decreased breathlessness and increased respiratory muscle endurance (Hamilton et al. 1995, Lisboa et al. 1994), but the benefits of inspiratory muscle strength training are not well established (Smith et al. 1992). Further research is needed to identify optimal candidates for respiratory muscle training and to clarify its benefits and role in pulmonary rehabilitation programmes.

Training reversibility

The reversibility of training effects is well known (American College of Sports Medicine 1986, Coyle et al. 1984). As with normal individuals, the training effects in patients with chronic lung disease are maintained only so long as exercise is continued. A reduction in adherence with the maintenance exercise prescription given at the completion of the formal pulmonary rehabilitation probably explains to some degree the reductions in timed walking distance (Vale et al. 1993) and exercise endurance time (Ries et al. 1995) occurring months to years later.

In a trial evaluating the long-term effects of home rehabilitation (Wijkstra et al. 1996), patients were randomized into three groups: a treatment group given 12 weeks of pulmonary rehabilitation followed by visits to a physical therapist once a week for a total of 18 months, another treatment group given the same formal rehabilitation but visited by the physical therapist once a month for 18 months, and a control group which received no rehabilitation at all but was followed for 18 months. Although both rehabilitation groups showed significant increased in maximal cycle workrate and 6-MWD post-rehabilitation, this improvement was not sustained at 18 months with either maintenance training frequency. There was an overall tendency for a decline in the 6-MWD after 18 months, but there were no significant difference between the two training frequencies. In another trial where patients completing formal rehabilitation were instructed to continue exercise training at home and to visit the programme once a month, the gains made in treadmill exercise endurance diminished considerably by 12 months (Ries et al. 1995). Neither of the above studies reported adherence with the post-rehabilitation exercise training. Thus, the optimal frequency and intensity of regular post-rehabilitation maintenance exercise training remains to be determined.

Additionally, the role of short periods of supervised exercise training following exacerbations of respiratory disease with a goal of returning the patient to baseline performance status is an untested alternative. Thus, although it is clear that efforts at improving long-term adherence with exercise training at home will be necessary for long-term effectiveness of pulmonary rehabilitation, further information from controlled trials is needed.

Dose response effect and maintenance

Health status measures and exercise performance following pulmonary rehabilitation are independently responsive to training, perhaps not surprisingly in view of the complexity of the former. Increases in exercise performance can occur quite quickly, but changes in health status may lag behind as patients gradually adjust to the lifestyle change. The optimum duration of physical training is unknown since direct comprehensive comparisons of the length of programmes have been published. One recent comparison suggests that improvements in physical performance occur by four weeks, but the improvements in health status may take longer (Green et al. 2001). The benefits of rehabilitation can be lasting but results of follow-up evaluation are mixed depending on factors such as intercurrent illness severity, etc. as a result of which performance indicators may decline (Singh et al. 1998, Cambach et al. 1999) despite best efforts to maintain progress made.

However, at least one-third of patients still retain significant improvements in health status after two years. There is no substantial evidence that prolonged maintenance treatment is beneficial or, if it is, what form it should take. However, the achievement of a more mobile lifestyle inclusive of the benefits of greater self-efficacy and confidence (Vogiatzis et al. 1999) are likely and certainly anecdotally reported by those patients who manage to progress to community- or sports-centre-based programmes.

Exercise and asthma

A number of studies have investigated fitness levels in asthmatic subjects. One study of 65 children with moderate to severe asthma revealed that 60 per cent were unfit and that 50 per cent were severely deconditioned (Ludwick et al. 1986). This was not simply a function of the severity of airways obstruction, as fitness levels could not be predicted from asthma history alone. Another large-scale study, again in children and using validated field testing of fitness by a nine-minute run (Strunk et al. 1988), showed poor conditioning (i.e. a score below the 25th percentile for values obtained from screening over 12,000 normal children) in 74 per cent of subjects that was not attributable to anthropometric differences. We used progressive incremental exercise testing (Clark and Cochrane 1988) not only to determine work performance but also to assess the contribution of respiratory factors to exercise limitation and to determine the likely capacity for endurance training in a group of patients with well-controlled asthma of moderate severity. Asthma accounted for a significant loss of fitness, but, contrary to the subjects' expectation, they achieved a maximum heart rate that was similar to that of control subjects and therefore had a normal cardiovascular rather than respiratory endpoint to exercise. We concluded that attitude to exercise was at least as important as disease severity in determining fitness in asthmatic adults.

Because asthma is a chronic illness that arises during early childhood, many long-standing misconceptions about the effect of exercise on the illness exist. There are few analogous conditions – for example angina and osteoarthritis – in which exercise has such a potentially deleterious effect on the patient not only by limiting exercise capability but also by acting as a direct stimulus to the underlying pathophysiological process. It is not surprising that asthmatic patients often have a negative attitude towards exercise. Whether the mechanism is respiratory heat loss (Deal et al. 1979) or increased osmolarity due to respiratory water loss (Sheppard and Eschenbacher 1984) or associated vascular events (McFadden 1990), increasing minute ventilation during exercise is a potent stimulus to exercise-induced asthma (EIA), which may occur as an isolated phenomenon or as an additional fall in airflow in the asthmatic patient with pre-existing obstruction. Fortunately, there is now a range of effective medications, including short- and long-acting beta-2 agonists and the newer leukotrienes, that can act prophylactically to prevent EIA and which are also prescribable under the rules of the International Olympic Committee. Pulmonary rehabilitation involves exercise under optimal conditions, with prior screening and medication and thus prevention of EIA with appropriate therapy as a prerequisite. Anderson et al. (1972) showed that treadmill exercise without prior treatment may produce an increase in ventilation/perfusion inequality, alveolo-arterial oxygen tension, physiological dead space and arterial blood lactate levels in addition to EIA – all of which can usually be effectively prevented with prior medication (Tan and Spector 1998).

However, many patients fall between the extremes of asthma severity, i.e. they have moderate airflow limitation despite medication. The pursuit of exercise as a recreational activity or as part of the widely advertised promotion of a healthy lifestyle raises a difficult question for these patients that is paradoxically not faced by severely disabled patients, namely how much exercise can and should be undertaken? At one extreme, the patient may attribute breathlessness to a lack of fitness when the illness is the limiting factor, and, at the other extreme, the patient may attribute exercise limitation to asthma despite good residual capacity for exercise participation.

Such objective information is not routinely available to the asthmatic patient, whose decision is heavily weighted against continuing to exercise whenever breathlessness is a significant component of the perceived exertion, regardless of its aetiology, because exercise in these circumstances may be viewed as potentially dangerous. One study (Meyer et al. 1990), by experimentally induced 'harmful anticipation', significantly intensified the perception of visceral changes, including the subjective cost of exercise, and even had some influence on specific asthma-related responses, such as airways resistance. There is evidence of a wide variability between exercise tolerance and measures of airways obstruction, as well as between the severity of breathlessness and measures of lung function in asthma (Mahler et al. 1991).

We have also reported beneficial changes in cardiorespiratory performance indicators in these asthmatic subjects following physical training using a carefully controlled programme of exercise training under medical supervision (Cochrane and Clark 1990). The three-month indoor training programme was carefully defined in terms of frequency, duration, intensity, progression and mode of physical activity. After training, there were significant increases in mean maximum oxygen uptake and anaerobic threshold. There were also significant reductions in blood lactate level, carbon dioxide production and VE at the higher levels of exercise in the training group. After training, breathlessness was also found to be reduced at workloads equivalent to those required by a wide range of daily activities. This confirms the general observation that patients with asthma may notice a diminution in symptoms (including breathlessness) after participating in an exercise programme (Haas et al. 1985).

In summary, patients with asthma should be considered for the same exercise options offered to patients with COPD but may constitute a more varied group in terms of illness severity and variability, age range and treatment requirements justifying provision of separate classes/sessions to take this into account

Use of oxygen during exercise training

Patients with normal oxygen tension at rest can show frequent and sometimes severe desaturation during activities of daily living (Schenkel et al. 1996), so the prescription of oxygen in rehabilitation is a difficult area. There is no consensus about identification of the need for supplemental oxygen or the optimal mode of delivery, but the routine use of supplemental oxygen in patients undergoing mild-exercise-induced desaturation does not enhance rehabilitation outcomes (Rooyackers et al. 1997, Garrod et al. 2000). Most published studies do not report oxygen usage but, for the present, it would be reasonable to recommend that supplementary oxygen be provided during exercise when clinically important desaturation (SpO_2 < 90 per cent) has been found at the training load in the preliminary test. Clearly, once ambulatory oxygen is recommended for training, it should be continued for similar activity at home, in line with the recent guidelines from the Royal College of Physicians (Royal College of Physicians 1999).

Facilities required for exercise programmes

There are two distinct modes of exercise programme requiring separate facilities: aerobic/mobility training and multigym weight training. Both can be supplemented by instruction to the patient to incorporate simple walking into their daily routine. This requires planning – i.e. tolerable distances and areas to walk need to be identified by the patient, and a log kept of progress in order to document fully the exercise being undertaken during pulmonary rehabilitation. Although programmes for aerobic/mobility training may vary, they require adequate floor space and heating, as provided in a typical indoor gymnasium. Unlike aerobics classes in healthy adults, however, the instructor not only supervises the group but also monitors each individual patient. The size of group at any session is therefore limited to eight to ten patients and the overall gym area need not be large (225 square metres is adequate). Multigym training uses specialized equipment to provide a circuit of exercises for individual muscle groups. A separate exercise area is essential, and again this need not be large, as there are the same constraints on patient numbers as already described. Each item of equipment may stand alone, but a combined multi-user apparatus containing up to eight items, with one or two extra stand-alone items to complete the requirements, provides for efficient use of limited space. A similar approach has recently improved endurance in patients with COPD. Cardiopulmonary resuscitation facilities with staff training are essential for all exercise programmes, although there have been no reports of significant critical incidents in the large and varied reports of pulmonary rehabilitation.

References

American College of Sports Medicine (1986) Guidelines for graded exercise testing and exercise prescription (third edition). Philadelphia, Pa: Lea and Febiger.

American College of Sports Medicine (2002) ACSM's exercise management for persons with chronic diseases and disabilities (second edition). Champaign, Ill: Human Kinetics.

American Thoracic Society (ATS) (1999) Pulmonary rehabilitation. American Journal of Respiratory and Critical Care Medicine 159: 166–182.

Anderson SD, Silverman M, Walker SR (1972) Metabolic and ventilatory changes in asthmatic patients during and after exercise. Thorax. 27(6): 718–725.

Astrand PO, Rhodahl K (2003) Textbook of work physiology: physiological bases of exercise (fourth edition). New York: McGraw-Hill.

Begin P, Grassino A (1991) Inspiratory muscle dysfunction and chronic hypercapnia in chronic obstructive pulmonary disease. American Review of Respiratory Disease 143(5 Part 1): 905–912.

Belman MJ, Kendregan BA (1982) Physical training fails to improve ventilatory muscle endurance in patients with chronic obstructive pulmonary disease. Chest 81(4): 440–443.

Black LF, Hyatt RE (1969) Maximal respiratory pressures: normal values and relationship to age and sex. American Review of Respiratory Disease 99(5): 696–702.

British Thoracic Society (BTS) (2001) Pulmonary rehabilitation. Thorax 56: 827–834.

Brown AB, McCartney N, Sale DG (1990) Positive adaptation to weightlifting training in the elderly. Journal of Applied Physiology 69: 1725–1733.

Cambach W, Chadwick-Straver RV, Wagenaar RC et al. (1997) The effects of a community-based pulmonary rehabilitation programme on exercise tolerance and quality of life: a randomized controlled trial. European Respiratory Journal 10(1): 104–113.

Cambach W, Wagenaar RC, Koelman TW et al. (1999) The long-term effects of pulmonary rehabilitation in patients with asthma and chronic obstructive pulmonary disease: a research synthesis Archives of Physical Medicine and Rehabilitation 80(1): 103–111.

Casaburi R, Patessio A, Loli F et al. (1991) Reductions in exercise lactic acidosis and ventilation as a result of exercise training in patients with obstructive lung disease. American Review of Respiratory Disease 143(1): 9–18.

Casaburi R, Porszasz J, Burns MR et al. (1997) Physiologic benefits of exercise training in rehabilitation of patients with severe chronic obstructive pulmonary disease. American Journal of Respiratory and Critical Care Medicine 155(5): 1541–1551.

Clark CJ, Cochrane LM (1988) Assessment of work performance in asthma for determination of cardiorespiratory fitness and training capacity. Thorax 43(10): 745–749.

Clark CJ, Cochrane L, Mackay E (1996) Low intensity peripheral muscle conditioning improves exercise tolerance and breathlessness in COPD. European Respiratory Journal 9(12): 2590–2596.

Clark CJ, Cochrane LM, Mackay E et al. (2000) Skeletal muscle strength and endurance in patients with mild COPD and the effects of weight training. European Respiratory Journal 15(4): 92–97.

Cochrane LM, Clark CJ (1990) Benefits and problems of a physical training programme for asthmatic patients. Thorax 45(5): 345–351.

Coyle EF, Martin WH, Sinacore DR et al. (1984) Time course of loss of adaptations after stopping prolonged intense endurance training. Journal of Applied Physiology 57(6): 1857–1864.

Deal EC, McFadden ER Jnr, Ingram RH et al. (1979) Role of respiratory heat exchange in the production of exercise-induced asthma. Journal of Applied Physiology 46(3): 467–475.

Debusk RF, Strnestrand U, Sheehan M et al. (1990) Training effects of long versus short bouts of exercise in healthy subjects. American Journal of Cardiology 65(15): 1010–1013.

Dekhuijzen PNR, Folgering HTM, van Herwaarden CLA (1991) Target-flow inspiratory muscle training during pulmonary rehabilitation in patients with COPD. Chest 99(1): 128–133.

Fernal B, Daniels FS (1984) Electroencephalographic changes after a prolonged running period: evidence for a relaxation response (abstract). Medicine and Science in Sports and Exercise 16: 181.

Garrod R, Paul EA, Wedzicha JA (2000) Supplemental oxygen during pulmonary rehabilitation in patients with COPD with exercise hypoxaemia. Thorax 55(7): 539–543.

Goldstein RS, Gort EH, Stubbing D et al. (1994) Randomised controlled trial of respiratory rehabilitation. Lancet 344(8934): 1394–1397.

Gosselink R, Wagenaar RC, Decramer M (1996) The reliability of a commercially available threshold loading device. Thorax 51(6): 601–605.

Green RH, Singh SJ, Williams J et al. (2001) A randomised controlled trial of four weeks versus seven weeks of pulmonary rehabilitation in chronic obstructive pulmonary disease Thorax 56(2): 143–145.

Haas FH, Pineda K, Axen D et al. (1985) Effects of physical fitness on expiratory airflow in exercising asthmatic people. Medicine and Science in Sports and Exercise 17(5): 585–592.

Hamilton AL, Killian KJ, Summers E et al. (1995) Muscle strength, symptom intensity, and exercise capacity in patients with cardiorespiratory disorders. American Journal of Respiratory and Critical Care Medicine 152(6 Part 1): 2021–2031.

Harver A, Mahler DA, Daubenspeck JA (1989) Targeted inspiratory muscle training improves respiratory muscle function and reduces dyspnea in patients with chronic obstructive pulmonary disease. Annals of Internal Medicine 111(2): 117–124.

Holloszy JO, Coyle EF (1984) Adaptations of skeletal muscle to endurance exercise and their metabolic consequences. Journal of Applied Physiology 56(4): 831–838.

Horowitz MB, Littenberg B, Mahler DA (1996) Dyspnea ratings for prescribing exercise intensity in patients with COPD. Chest 109(5): 1169–1175.

Jones NL (1997) Clinical Exercise Testing (fourth edition). Philadelphia, Pa: WB Saunders & Company.

Katch VL, Weltman A, Sady S et al. (1978) Validity of the relative percent concept for equating training intensity. European Journal of Applied Physiology and Occupational Physiology 39(4): 219–227.

Killian KJ, Jones NL (1988) Respiratory muscles and dyspnea. Clinics in Chest Medicine 9(2): 237–248.

Kim MJ, Larson JL, Covey MK et al. (1993) Inspiratory muscle training in patients with chronic obstructive pulmonary disease. Nursing Research 42(6): 356–362.

Lake FR, Henderson K, Briffa T et al. (1990) Upper-limb and lower-limb exercise training in patients with chronic airflow obstruction. Chest 97(5): 1077–1082.

Larson JL, Kim MJ, Sharp JT et al. (1988) Inspiratory muscle training with a pressure threshold breathing device in patients with chronic obstructive pulmonary disease. American Review of Respiratory Disease 138: 689–696.

Lisboa C, Munoz V, Beroiza T et al. (1994) Inspiratory muscle training in chronic airflow limitation: comparison of two different training loads with a threshold device. European Respiratory Journal 7: 1266–1274.

Ludwick SK, Jones JW, Jones TK et al. (1986) Normalisation of cardiopulmonary endurance in severely asthmatic children after bicycle ergometry therapy. Journal of Pediatrics 109: 446–451.

Mahler DA, Cunningham LN, Skrinar GS et al. (1989) Activity and hypercapnic ventilatory responsiveness after marathon running. Journal of Applied Physiology 66(5): 2431–2437.

Mahler DA, Faryniarz K, Lentine T et al. (1991) Measurement of breathlessness during exercise in asthmatics. Predictor variables, reliability and responsiveness. American Review of Respiratory Disease 144(1): 39–44.

Maltais F, LeBlanc P, Simard C et al. (1996) Skeletal muscle adaptation to endurance training in patients with chronic obstructive pulmonary disease. American Journal of Respiratory and Critical Care Medicine 154(2 Part 1): 442–447.

Maltais F, LeBlanc P, Jobin J et al. (1997) Intensity of training and physiologic adaptation in patients with chronic obstructive pulmonary disease. American Journal of Critical Care Medicine 155: 555–561.

Martinez FJ, Vogel PD, Dupont DN et al. (1993) Supported arm exercise vs. unsupported arm exercise in the rehabilitation of patients with severe chronic airflow obstruction. Chest 103(5): 1397–1402.

McFadden ER Jr (1990) Exercise-induced asthma as a vascular phenomenon. Lancet 335: 880–883.

Meyer R, Kroner-Herwig B, Sporkel H (1990) The effect of exercise and induced expectations on visceral perception in asthmatic patients. Journal of Psychosomatic Research 34(4): 455–460.

O'Donnell DE, McGuire MA, Samis L et al. (1995) The impact of exercise reconditioning on breathlessness in severe chronic airflow limitation. American Journal of Critical Care Medicine 152(6 Part 1): 2005–2013.

Poole DC, Gaesser GA (1985) Response of ventilatory and lactate thresholds to continuous and interval training. Journal of Applied Physiology 58(4): 1115–1221.

Punzal PA, Ries AL, Kaplan RM et al. (1991) Maximum intensity exercise training in patients with chronic obstructive pulmonary disease. Chest 100(3): 618–623.

Ries AL, Kaplan RM, Limberg TM et al. (1995) Effects of pulmonary rehabilitation on physiologic and psychosocial outcomes in patients with chronic obstructive pulmonary disease. Annals of Internal Medicine 122(11): 823–832.

Rooyackers JM, Dekhuijzen PN, van Herwaarden CL et al. (1997) Training with supplemental oxygen in patients with COPD and hypoxaemia at peak exercise. European Respiratory Journal 10(6): 1278–1284.

Royal College of Physicians (1999) Domiciliary oxygen therapy services: clinical guidelines and advice for prescribers. Report of a working party. London: Royal College of Physicians.

Schenkel NS, Burdet L, de Muralt B et al. (1996) Oxygen saturation during daily activities in chronic obstructive pulmonary disease. European Respiratory Journal 9(12): 2584–2589.

Schols AMWJ, Coppoolse R, Akkermans M et al. (1996) Physiological effects of interval versus endurance training in patients with severe COPD (abstract). American Journal of Critical Care Medicine 153: A127.

Sheppard D, Eschenbacher WL (1984) Respiratory water loss as a stimulus to exercise-induced bronchoconstriction. Journal of Allergy and Clinical Immunology 73: 640–642.

Simpson K, Killian K, McCartney N et al. (1992) Randomised controlled trial of weightlifting exercise in patients with chronic airflow limitation. Thorax 47(2): 70–75.

Singh SJ, Smith DL, Hyland ME et al. (1998) A short outpatient pulmonary rehabilitation programme: immediate and longer-term effects on exercise performance and quality of life. Respiratory Management 92(9): 1146–1154.

Smith K, Cook K, Guyatt GH et al. (1992) Respiratory muscle training in chronic airflow obstruction. American Review of Respiratory Disease 145: 533–539.

Stark RD (1988) Dyspnoea: assessment and pharmacological manipulation. European Respiratory Journal 1(3): 280–287.

Strunk RC, Rubin D, Kelly L et al. (1988) Determination of fitness in children with asthma. Use of standardised tests for functional endurance, body fat composition, flexibility and abdominal strength. American Journal of Diseases of Children 142(9): 940–944.

Tan RA, Spector SL (1998) Exercise-induced asthma (review). Sports Medicine 25: 1–6.

Vale F, Reardon JZ, ZuWallack RL (1993) The long-term benefits of outpatient pulmonary rehabilitation on exercise endurance and quality of life. Chest 103(1): 42–45.

Vallet G, Ahmaidi S, Serres I et al. (1997) Comparison of two training programmes in chronic airway limitation patients: standardized versus individualized protocols. European Respiratory Journal 10(1): 114–122.

Vogiatzis I, Williamson AF, Miles J et al. (1999) Physiological response to moderate exercise workloads in a pulmonary rehabilitation programme in patients with varying degrees of airflow obstruction. Chest 116(5): 1200–1207.

Wasserman K, Hansen JE, Sue DY et al. (1994) Pathophysiology of disorders limiting exercise. In: Principles of Exercise Testing and Interpretation (second edition). Philadelphia: Lea and Febiger.

Wijkstra PJ, van der Mark TW, Kraan J et al. (1996) Effects of home rehabilitation on physical performance in patients with chronic obstructive pulmonary disease (COPD). European Respiratory Journal 9(1): 104–110.

Chapter 5
Assessment of exercise performance and muscle function in pulmonary rehabilitation

R. GOSSELINK, T. TROOSTERS, M. DECRAMER

Introduction

In patients with chronic obstructive pulmonary disease (COPD), dyspnoea, impaired exercise tolerance and reduced quality of life are common complaints. Several pieces of evidence point to the fact that these features are not simply consequences of the loss of pulmonary function. Reduced exercise capacity shows only a weak relation to lung function impairment (Wasserman et al. 1989). Prediction of exercise performance based on resting pulmonary function tests is inaccurate (McGavin et al. 1976, Morgan et al. 1983, Swinburn et al. 1985). Other factors, such as respiratory and peripheral-muscle weakness, deconditioning and impaired gas exchange, may also contribute to reduced exercise tolerance. Reduced muscle strength in COPD is observed both for respiratory (Decramer et al. 1980, Perez et al. 1996, Rochester and Braun 1985) and peripheral muscles (Decramer et al. 1994, Gosselink et al. 1996, Hamilton et al. 1995). Muscle atrophy is substantiated (Gosselink et al. 1996, Hamilton et al. 1995) by reductions of muscle cross-sectional area (Bernard et al. 1998) and muscle fibre cross-sectional area (Whittom et al. 1998). The importance of peripheral skeletal muscle weakness to the impairment of exercise capacity in patients with COPD was demonstrated by several authors (Gosselink et al. 1996, Killian et al. 1992) and in detail described in a recent overview (Casaburi 2001). Quadriceps force contributes significantly to six-minute walking distance (6-MWD) and maximal oxygen uptake (Gosselink et al. 1996, Hamilton et al. 1995). Indeed, a significant reduction in muscle strength was observed after high-intensity exercise in COPD patients (Mador et al. 2000), further substantiating the role of muscle weakness in exercise limitation. Respiratory muscle weakness contributes to hypercapnia (Begin and Grassino 1991), dyspnoea (Hamilton, et al. 1995, Killian and Jones 1988), nocturnal oxygen desaturation (Heijdra et al. 1996) and to reduced walking distance (Gosselink et al. 1996).

In addition, muscle weakness contributes to utilization of health care resources (Decramer et al. 1997), and peripheral muscle strength as well as skeletal muscle atrophy were shown to be significant determinants of survival in patients with COPD (Decramer et al. 1998, Decramer et al. 1996, Marquis et al. 2002).

Prior to a respiratory rehabilitation programme, exercise performance has to be investigated for a diagnosis of impaired exercise capacity, identification of factors limiting exercise performance, and the prescription of exercise training. This chapter will deal with various modalities of exercise testing, and tests for respiratory and peripheral muscle function.

Exercise testing

Ergometry is performed to assess exercise capacity to answer the question of whether exercise capacity is impaired and what the causes of exercise limitation are. Unexplained dyspnoea during exercise is a frequent reason for exercise testing, more specific for respiratory rehabilitation (Casaburi et al. 1991) and exercise-induced asthma (Folgering et al. 1987). The reason for exercise testing should be specified, and accordingly the appropriate type of exercise and protocol should be chosen. A patient may be referred for exercise testing for functional assessment or for a follow-up of interventions, such as respiratory rehabilitation (Solway et al. 2001). In these cases, valuable clinical information is easily obtained from constant workrate tests or walking tests (shuttle walking tests or timed walking tests). Sub-maximal exercise 'field' tests, like the 6- or 12-MWD (McGavin et al. 1976), shuttle run test or shuttle walk test (Singh et al. 1992) and step tests, are easy to perform and seem valid tests since they are more related to activities of daily living. For some of these tests, however, the lack of reference values and the absence of physiological measures are important limitations of the test. In healthy subjects, a fairly good correlation with VO_2max is observed, but not good enough to predict VO_2max in individuals (Astrand 1960, Froelicher et al. 1974, Froelicher et al. 1975).

Sub-maximal exercise testing – field tests and endurance tests

Six- (or 12-) MWD

In this test, functional exercise capacity is expressed in meters covered by the patient in six or 12 minutes (Guyatt et al. 1984, McGavin et al. 1976). This popular test was reported to be done in approximately 80 per cent of the rehabilitation programmes in the USA (Stevens et al. 1999). The test is performed in a corridor with a known track length. Patients are instructed to cover as many meters as possible in the scheduled time. If needed, patients are allowed to have rest periods during the test, to restart and change the walking speed. At the end of the test, patients must have the feeling of a maximal test. Besides the distance covered, also heart rate, transcutaneous oxygen saturation (StcO$_2$) and Borg Symptom Scale ratings for dyspnoea and fatigue are taken at the end of the exercise test. All these measures give additional information (van Stel et al. 2001).

Encouragement is standardized, and the test has to be repeated at least once (Guyatt et al. 1984). Further repetitions of the test results in only limited progression of the test result (~3 per cent). A recent guideline published by the American Thoracic Society stresses the importance of proper standardization (ATS 2002b). To ensure reproducible and reliable results, the following guidelines are proposed:

- Prepare written-down instructions for all staff members involved in performing timed-walking tests (this should also include the spoken instruction given to the patient prior to the test).
- Standardize the encouragement during the test in terms of phrases used and timing (every 30 seconds, encouragement can be given to maximize patient's effort).
- Record oxygen saturation, heart rate and symptoms – use validated Borg Symptom Scale (0–10) to assess symptoms of dyspnoea and fatigue.
- Supplementary oxygen is provided during the test when necessary (the investigator carries oxygen).
- Repeat the test at least once after sufficient rest (30–60 minutes).

The availability of normal values (Enright and Sherrill 1998, Troosters et al. 1999b, Pardy et al. 1981) and minimal clinically relevant difference (54 m), for the 6-WMD (Redelmeier et al. 1997), has contributed to the interpretability of the data. In addition, a recent study described the physiological load during a six-minute walking test (Troosters et al. 2002). The 6-WMD proved to be a strenuous, constant workrate test. The test is therefore perfectly suited to investigate the effects of interventions that alter endurance capacity, like respiratory rehabilitation, and give information that is complementary to information obtained during incremental exercise testing. This chapter highlights an important safety issue. Oxygen desaturation, hypercapnia, oxygen consumption and heart rate are largely identical to what is obtained during incremental exercise testing. It should be stressed that investigators are trained in detecting alarm symptoms that may occur during this field exercise test (pallor, angina, dizziness, extreme dyspnoea) and are trained in basic life-saving procedures.

Incremental shuttle walking test

The incremental shuttle walking test is an incremental, externally paced exercise test that stresses the patient to a symptom-limited maximum (Singh et al. 1992). The patient walks around a ten-meter course, defined by two marker cones. The speed of walking is dictated by signals played from a tape cassette and increases every minute until the patient is unable to keep up with the speed due to breathlessness or fatigue. The walking distance correlates well with VO_2max (Singh et al. 1994) but, to date, no reference values are available. As this is a maximal incremental exercise test, the results obtained with this test may overlap with those obtained during an incremental ergometer test.

Cycle endurance test

In the follow-up of patients after respiratory rehabilitation and medication, constant workrate tests performed on a bicycle or treadmill were shown to be sensitive (O'Donnell et al. 1998, O'Donnell and Webb 1998). Test–retest reliability is good (van 't Hul et al. 2003). These tests, however, require at least one maximal incremental exercise test preceding the consecutive follow-up tests. The follow-up tests are made at a fixed workrate (70 per cent of the peak workrate of the preceding incremental test) (Goldstein et al. 1994, Simpson et al. 1992). The power output that can be sustained (theoretically) for ever is called the *critical power*. No data are available on normal values, but the critical power in normal subjects is around 70 per cent of the peak workload (Neder et al. 2000). Nevertheless, the data obtained from a constant workrate test are of physiological relevance. These tests can vary in complexity from analysis of exercise time, ventilation, heart rate and symptom scores to the analysis of the organ system responses at the onset of exercise. Oxygen uptake, carbon dioxide production, ventilation and heart rate responses are characterized by a time constant (τ). This is the time needed to reach 63 per cent of the final steady state change (Whipp et al. 1998). The oxygen uptake kinetics in this test reflects the overall oxidative capacity of the muscles (including capillarization, muscle fibres, oxidative enzymes) and, in COPD, seems to be influenced by the oxygen delivery to the working muscles (Palange et al. 1995). This last approach is reserved for research situations, and standardization is critical to obtain reliable results.

Endurance shuttle walking test

This test is based on the incremental shuttle walking test. The patient is asked to sustain walking as long as possible at a speed obtained at 85 per cent of the maximal walking speed during the shuttle walking test (after a practice shuttle walk) (Revill et al. 1999). Walking speed during the endurance shuttle walking test is dictated by signals played from a tape cassette. The test will be terminated when the patient is, for the second consecutive lap, unable to get to the cone in the preset time. Good reproducibility is obtained after one practice walking test. The endurance shuttle walking test seems to be more sensitive to changes after respiratory rehabilitation than the shuttle walking test (Revill et al. 1999).

Maximal exercise testing

The gold standard in exercise testing is the incremental exercise test. The introduction of computerized breath-by-breath equipment made the test available to most clinical settings. Incremental exercise testing is the first choice when assessing impaired exercise capacity to investigate the factors limiting exercise performance, to assess risk in participating in exercise programmes or to prescribe exercise training. For all these indications, incremental exercise testing is necessary to provide clinicians with key data that cannot be obtained from resting measures of pulmonary function, cardiac function, blood gases, functional exercise tests or constant work-rate tests.

Ergometer (treadmill or bicycle) tests

For incremental exercise testing, two ergometers can be selected: a treadmill and a cycle ergometer. When a motor-driven treadmill is used, increasing the speed and/or the inclination of the treadmill imposes the external workload. Compared to cycling, a larger amount of muscle mass is put to work, which results in 5 to 10 per cent higher VO_2peak. Therefore, standardized maximal exercise tests were developed (Astrand and Saltin 1961, Hermansen and Saltin 1969, McArdle et al. 1973). On a bicycle ergometer, the workload is better controlled and the external work is less dependent on body weight. Bicycle ergometry, unlike treadmill ergometry, allows the investigator to compare patients' responses to iso sub-maximal work and allows clearer insight into mechanical efficiency. Factors such as walking efficiency (depending on footwear, length of the lower limb and training status on treadmills) and the use of arm support may have an unpredictable influence on the VO_2 profile during treadmill testing. The stability of the patient on a bicycle results in less noise in the ECG signal and blood-pressure data. In addition, the access to arterial or venous catheters is easier on a cycle ergometer. Cycle ergometers for exercise testing should be electromagnetically braked and should have the ability to adjust the workload in 5 to 10 Watt steps.

Exercise protocol

An incremental exercise test consists of baseline measurements of at least two to three minutes, then a warm-up period of three minutes' unloaded pedalling, followed by the incremental part of the exercise test. When peak exercise is reached, patients will continue cycling for some minutes at a very low work-rate to avoid a sudden drop in blood pressure due to a venous pooling of blood. The choice of the adequate increment size is one of the important steps in the design of the exercise test and in the tailoring of the test to the individual patient. Ideally, peak workrate is reached within eight to 12 minutes. Several authors have suggested prediction equations for workrate increments. The workrate increments have important consequences when the incremental exercise results are used to target the training intensity in a pulmonary rehabilitation programme. Different increment sizes do not affect peak oxygen uptake, ventilation or heart rate (Debigare et al. 2000). Peak workrate, however, varies significantly between different protocols, being higher in 'steeper' protocols (protocols with larger increments). Consequently, this may affect the exercise prescription, as it is frequently based on peak workrate. When patients are tested consecutively, the increment size should be kept unchanged.

Measurements

In clinical practice, measurements are workrate, 12-lead electro-cardiography, blood pressure, pulmonary gas exchange (VO_2 and VCO_2), pulmonary ventilation, transcutaneous oxygen saturation and symptom scores. When arterial blood gases are available at rest and peak exercise, most clinical problems regarding exercise limitations can be addressed. Symptom scores for dyspnoea and exertion have been shown to be valuable tools during exercise testing. Visual analogue scales and Borg Breathlessness Scales cannot be interchanged, but both show good agreement and hence are valid tools to evaluate symptoms of dyspnoea and perceived exertion (Wilson and Jones 1991). A number of texts are available to aid the interpretation of exercise testing (Jones et al. 1985, Wasserman et al. 1994). Variables at sub-maximal exercise and at peak exercise are integrated to answer questions on exercise capacity, safety of exercise, and limitation of exercise, and specific questions like exercise prescription. It is important that the protocol of the exercise tests takes into account the clinical and medical history of the patient.

Physical exercise capacity of the patient

The main outcome of the maximal exercise test is maximal oxygen uptake, standardized per kilogram of body weight. A comparison with reference values allows judging on the level of exercise impairment. The European Respiratory Society report on exercise impairment in patients with respiratory disease (Cotes 1990) reported on two equations for reference values for VO_2max. The equation of Jones et al. (1985) seems useful in clinical practice for cycle aerometry (Table 5.1). Exercise labs should be encouraged to test some healthy control subjects in the age span of interest to evaluate which normal values suit their laboratory best.

In a physiological sense, the exercise is maximal when one or more components related to oxygen transport or muscle-force generation are maximally loaded. Pulmonary gas exchange, ventilation, circulation and muscle function (including peripheral gas exchange) are considered to be the components of the oxygen transport chain. In addition, intolerable symptoms mostly terminate exercise performance. Killian et al. (1992) found that Borg scores of 7 to 8 were perceived as unacceptable symptoms.

Table 5.1 Reference values for maximal oxygen uptake

$0.046 \times H - 0.021 \times A - 0.62 \times S - 4.31$ (SD: 0.458)	male and female	(Jones et al. 1985)
$W \times (50.7 - 0.372 \times A)$ $(50.7 - 0.372 \times A) + \{6 \times (W\text{-}Wnl)\}$ $\{(Wnl + W)/2\} \times (50.7 - 0.372 \times A)$ predicted normal weight (Wnl) = $0.65 \times H - 42.8$	male overweight underweight	(Wasserman et al. 1994)
$(W + 43) \times (22.78 - 0.17 \times H)$ $(W + 43) \times (22.78 - 0.17 \times A) + \{6 \times (W\text{-}Wnl)\}$ $\{(Wnl + W + 86)/2\} \times (22.78 - 0.17 \times age)$ predicted normal weight (Wnl) = $0.65 \times H - 42.8$	female overweight underweight	(Wasserman et al. 1994)

VO_2l/min., H = height in cm, W = weight in kg, Wnl = predicted normal weight in kg, A = age, S = gender, male = 0, female = 1

Causes of exercise limitation

Exercise performance will be limited by the weakest component of the physiological chain of ventilation, pulmonary gas exchange, muscle cell metabolism, muscle force and perception of fatigue and dyspnoea (Dempsey 1986, Wasserman et al. 1994). More specifically the following limitations might be identified (Table 5.2):

Table 5.2 Causes of exercise limitation

	PaO_2	$PaCO_2$	$D(A\text{-}a)O_2$	HR	VEmax	PIplmax PEplmax	Borg score D/E
Cardiocirc. limitation	=	↓	<2kPa	>HRmax	<MVV	not reached	↑E
V/Q mismatch	↓/=	=	↑/=	<HRmax	<MVV	not reached	↑D
Ventilatory limitation	↓	↑	<2kPa	<HRmax	>70%MVV	possibly reached	↑D
Pulmonary gas exchange	↓	=	>2kPa	<HRmax	<MVV	possibly reached	↑D
Peripheral muscle weakness	=	=	<2kPa	<HRmax	<MVV	not reached	↑↑E
Psychogenic limitation	=	=	<2kPa	<HRmax	<MVV	not reached	↑↑D

$D(A\text{-}a)O_2$ = alveolar-arterial oxygen difference, V/Q = ventilation-perfusion mismatch, HR = heart rate at maximal exercise, HR max = 220 – age (years) (predicted maximal heart rate), VEmax = maximal minute ventilation, MVV = maximal voluntary ventilation, PIplmax = maximal inspiratory pleural pressure, PEplmax = maxima expiratory pleural pressure, D = dyspnoea-sensation, E = exertion, = no change, ↑ increase, ↓ decrease

A *cardiocirculatory limitation* is identified when cardiac output fails to increase in order to meet the required oxygen delivery. Heart rate assessment is used as a non-invasive indicator of cardiac output. Achievement of the age-specific maximal heart rate (220 – age +/– 10 beats/ min) is indicative of the maximum cardiac output. This limitation is observed in healthy subjects, and frequently in patients with an FEV_1 larger than 50 per cent predicted (Dekhuijzen et al. 1991). This exercise limitation is not a direct consequence of the pulmonary disease. In other conditions, like heart failure or ischemia, the maximal heart rate may not be reached, but a low ratio of VO_2/HR and high sub-maximal heart rates, together with other findings (echocardiography, ECG changes), may help to interpret a cardiocirculatory limitation.

A *ventilatory limitation* is related to an imbalance between the load and capacity of the respiratory pump. The load on the pump is increased due to airway obstruction altered lung/chest-wall compliance. The capacity of the ventilatory pump might be impaired due to respiratory muscle weakness (Efthimiou et al. 1988) and reduced ventilatory drive. A ventilatory limitation is frequently observed in patients with more advanced lung disease, and airway obstruction (FEV_1 < 50 per cent pred), chest wall deformities, respiratory muscle weakness and in patients with interstitial lung disease and neuromuscular disease. A ventilatory limitation can be identified in different ways. An increase in arterial PCO_2 during the exercise test can be observed, but this response might strongly be influenced by the central drive. Second, minute ventilation that exceeds 70–80 per cent of the maximal voluntary ventilation (MVV ~$37.5 \times FEV_1$) is considered a ventilatory limitation. More recently, inspections of the tidal flow-volume loop during exercise were shown to be useful in the interpretation of ventilatory limitation, especially to assess dynamic hyperinflation during exercise (reducing the capacity of the ventilatory pump), measurements of inspiratory capacity or flow-volume loops may be useful (O'Donnell 2002).

Pulmonary gas exchange limitation is identified by an isolated reduction in arterial PO_2 and/or an increase in the alveolar-arterial oxygen gradient of greater than 2kPa (Wasserman et al. 1994). It is unclear why these patients stop exercise. Some patients do not sense hypoxemia and continue exercise up to very low values of PaO_2, while other patients stop exercise when PaO_2 has hardly decreased (Mak et al. 1993). Exercise tests will be terminated by the investigator when oxygen saturation drops below 80 per cent. A low T_{Lco} has some prediction for exercise-induced hypoxemia (Wijkstra et al. 1994). In the absence of significant airflow limitation, T_{Lco} values below 50 per cent predicted will cause hypoxemia in most patients. During exercise in more severe COPD, ventilation-perfusion inhomogeneity will decrease, while diffusion will deteriorate. The net effect will be that PaO_2 and (A-a)DO_2 do not alter (Agusti et al. 1990).

In addition, *peripheral muscle weakness* might also contribute to reduced exercise capacity (Gosselink et al. 1996) (see below in detail). At the end of the exercise test, patients rate their level of exertion with the

Borg score for leg exertion high. Additional muscle-strength measurements of leg and arm muscles are needed to further explore muscle weakness as the limiting factor of exercise performance. Peripheral gas exchange problems are more difficult to address. In clinical routine testing, complaints of pain may be suggestive of peripheral gas exchange limitation.

Finally, psychological factors, such as fear, anxiety or lack of motivation, can also contribute to low exercise performance. A psychological limitation is concluded when no other limitations of exercise performance can be identified, as pointed out above.

Muscle testing

Assessment of skeletal muscle function contributes to the evaluation of impairment of COPD patients and thus to the assessment of rehabilitation in several ways. Skeletal muscle function is an independent marker of disease severity (Marquis, et al. 2002) since it contributes to the above-mentioned clinically relevant issues. Muscle-function assessment enables the health care professional to diagnose muscle weakness and thus to state the indication for rehabilitation. Indeed, isometric muscle testing seems helpful in selecting candidates for exercise training in healthy subjects (Wilson and Murphy 1996) and in COPD patients (Troosters et al. 2001). COPD patients with muscle weakness seem to be better responders to rehabilitation (Troosters et al. 2001). The measurement of isometric muscle strength and endurance was also found to be sensitive when detecting changes in peripheral muscle function after rehabilitation (O'Donnell et al. 1998, Simpson et al. 1992, Troosters et al. 1996a, Troosters et al. 1996b, Troosters et al. 2000b).

Skeletal muscle strength is in general reduced in COPD. However, arm-muscle strength is less affected than leg-muscle and respiratory-muscle strength (Bernard et al. 1998, Gosselink et al. 2000), while proximal arm muscles were more affected than distal arm and hand muscles (Gosselink et al. 2000). This information is helpful to optimize training prescription in a rehabilitation programme, which allows health care professionals to target muscle training so that it is more specific to more impaired muscle groups.

The assessment of respiratory and peripheral skeletal muscle function will be discussed from the point of view of both strength and endurance capacity of the muscles.

Peripheral muscle strength testing

Muscle strength – or, more precisely, the maximum muscle force or tension generated by a muscle or (mostly) a group of muscles – can be measured in several ways and with different equipment. Manual testing with the 0–5 scale from the Medical Research Council is often used in clinical practice but is very insensitive to assess differences in muscle strength of values above grade 3 (active movement against gravity). Therefore, the following equipment was developed to measure muscle strength more accurately:

1. One-repetition maximum (1-RM) weightlifting for isotonic muscle force is a dynamic method for measuring the maximum amount of weight lifted at one time during a standard weightlifting exercise. To achieve the maximum lift capacity, weight increments between 1 kg and 5 kg are used with intervals of 1 to 5 minutes between attempts. In elderly people, 1-RM can be calculated from sub-maximal efforts (Braith et al. 1993). For untrained persons the calculated 1 – RM (kg) = 1.554 × (7 – 10RM weight, kg) – 5.181. The 7 – 10RM weight represents approximately 68 per cent of the 1-RM score. For trained persons the calculated 1-RM (kg) = 1.172 × (7 – 10RM weight, kg) + 7.704. The 7 – 10RM weight represents approximately 79 per cent of the 1-RM score. In COPD patients, the 1-RM tests have been shown to be safe (Kaelin et al. 1999) and sensitive to measure changes after training (Simpson et al. 1992). However, to the best of our knowledge, no normative data exist for the 1-RM tests, and the values obtained are largely dependent on the equipment used. Measurement of the 1-RM is often used to guide a muscle-training programme (Frontera et al. 1988, Frontera et al. 1990).
2. Dynamometry with mechanical or electrical equipment is used to measure isometric muscle force. In mechanical equipment mostly a steel spring is compressed, which moves a pointer on a scale, for example the handgrip dynamometer (Mathiowetz et al. 1985) (Figure 5.1). Handgrip dynamometry has been shown to be reliable, and reference values are available (Mathiowetz et al. 1984, Mathiowetz et al. 1985)

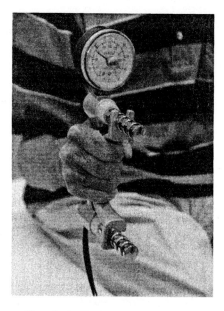

Figure 5.1 Assessment of handgrip force.

Table 5.3 Reference values for handgrip strength (Mathiowetz et al. 1985)

Age	Side	MALE Mean	Stand. dev	FEMALE Mean	Stand. dev
22–24	R	55	10	32	7
	L	48	10	28	6
25–29	R	55	10	34	6
	L	50	7	29	5
30–34	R	56	10	36	9
	L	50	10	31	8
35–39	R	55	11	34	5
	L	51	10	30	5
40–44	R	53	10	32	6
	L	51	9	28	6
45–49	R	50	10	28	7
	L	46	10	25	6
50–54	R	52	8	30	5
	L	46	8	26	5
55–59	R	46	12	26	6
	L	38	10	21	5
60–64	R	41	9	25	5
	L	37	9	21	5
65–69	R	41	10	23	5
	L	35	9	19	4
70–74	R	35	10	23	5
	L	30	8	19	5
75+	R	30	10	20	5
	L	25	8	17	4

(Table 5.3). It has been used in several studies in COPD patients (Gosselink et al. 1996, Kutsuzawa et al. 1992, Kutsuzawa et al. 1995, Wilson et al. 1986).

For other upper- and lower-extremity muscle groups hand-held devices have been developed. This electrical equipment consists of an electronic force transducer connected to a computer (Figure 5.2). Two methods of isometric testing are described: the *make-test* and the *break-test*. In the make-test, the maximal force of the subject is equal to the force of the observer. In the break-test, the force of the examiner exceeds the force of the patient slightly. Both tests are reproducible, but higher values were found during break-tests (Stratford and Balsor 1994). Hand-held dynamometry is a viable alternative to more costly modes of isometric strength measurements, provided the assessor's strength is greater than that of the specific muscle group being measured (Stratford and Balsor 1994, Troosters et al. 2000a). Reference values are available for elderly healthy subjects as well (Andrews et al. 1996, Phillips et al. 2000, van der Ploeg et al. 1991) (Table 5.4). Hand-held devices for muscle testing have been applied in COPD patients (Gosselink et al. 2000, Troosters et al. 1999a).

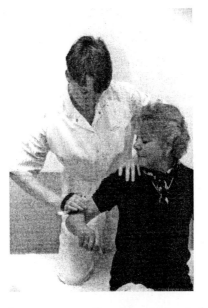

Figure 5.2 Position for the assessment of peripheral muscle force with hand-held dynamometry.

Table 5.4 Reference values for isometric muscle strength assessed with hand-held dynamometry (Andrews et al. 1996)

HAND-HELD DYNAMOMETRY

Knee extension (sitting upright, hip and knee 90° flexion)
$Y = 358.455 - 87.581 \times S + 2.914 \times W - 3.136 \times A$

Knee flexion (sitting upright, hip and knee 90° flexion)
$Y = 142.244 - 52.112 \times S + 1.85 \times W - 0.892 \times A$

Shoulder abduction (supine, shoulder 45° abduction, elbow 90° flexion)
$Y = 198.341 - 68.686 \times S + 1.324 \times W - 1.462 \times A$

Elbow flexion (supine, shoulder 15° abduction, elbow 90° flexion, supination)
$Y = 229.421 - 84.836 \times S + 1.618 \times W - 1.503 \times A$

Elbow extension (supine, shoulder 15° abduction, elbow 90° flexion, supination)
$Y = 112.597 - 49.858 \times S + 1.364 \times W - 0.834 \times A$

S= sex (0 = male, 1 = female), W = weight (in kg), A = age (in year), Y = strength

3. Computer-assisted dynamometers to measure isokinetic or isometric muscle strength have the advantage of measuring maximal muscle strength over a wide range of joint positions and velocities (Figure 5.3). This also takes into account the force-velocity characteristics of the muscle contraction. However, the equipment is very expensive and not available to many practitioners. Reference values are available for isometric (Decramer et al. 1996) and isotonic (Neder et al. 1999) muscle

testing. In healthy subjects, isometric and isokinetic measurements were well correlated (Borges 1989, Lord et al. 1992). Although direct comparison between these measures was not performed in COPD patients, two studies may suggest such a relationship also in COPD. Both isokinetic muscle strength (Clark et al. 2000, Hamilton et al. 1995) and isometric muscle strength (Decramer et al. 1994, Gosselink et al. 1996) were significantly lower in COPD patients compared to healthy subjects.

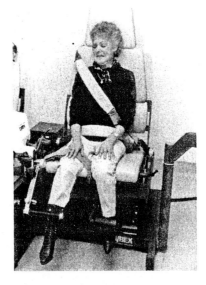

Figure 5.3 Positioning for the assessment of peripheral muscle strength with computer-assisted dynamometry.

The limitation of the use of maximal voluntary contractions is the potential to observe sub-maximal contractions due to sub-maximal cortical drive (Allen et al. 1995, Polkey et al. 1996). The use of superimposed electric or magnetic twitch contractions anticipates this potential variation in voluntary activation (Allen et al. 1995). The technique of electrically superimposed twitch contractions was developed in 1954 by Merton (Merton 1954). Twitch stimulation, however, is not suggested for routine clinical evaluation of muscle force. When standardized, and maximal encouragement is given, isometric muscle strength results in reliable and maximal data (Polkey et al. 1996).

Peripheral muscle endurance testing

The evaluation of lower-limb muscle performance in patients with COPD has focused mainly on muscle strength. In addition to reduced muscle fibre cross-sectional area (Whittom et al. 1998) and muscle cross-sectional area (Bernard et al. 1998), changes in fibre type composition resulting in a decrement of fatigue-resistant slow fibres (Evans et al. 1997, Jakobsson et al. 1990, Whittom et al. 1998) and a reduction in oxidative enzymes (Maltais et al. 1996, Maltais et al. 1998, Payen et al. 1993) are the main morphological and histochemical alterations found in lower-limb skeletal muscles. Following these morphological and histochemical alterations in muscle biopsies, it may be hypothesized that lower-limb muscle endurance is decreased more than muscle strength in patients with COPD. Newell et al. (1989) observed only a slight reduction in endurance capacity (torque reduction over 18 contractions) of elbow flexors in COPD patients compared to healthy subjects. The same was concluded for triceps and deltoid sustained contractions, which were not different between healthy subjects and patients with mild COPD (Clark et al. 2000). Along the same lines, endurance (time to maintain 80 per cent of peak torque) of the quadriceps muscle in hypoxemic COPD patients was normal (Zattara-Hartmann et al. 1995). In contrast, Serres et al. found a mean reduction of 50 per cent in quadriceps muscle endurance (number of contractions made at sub-maximal 20 to 40 per cent of peak torque) in patients with moderate to severe COPD (Serres et al. 1998). Van 't Hul et al. (2004) observed a reduction of 70 to 80 per cent of the endurance capacity of the quadriceps muscle in COPD.

Isolated muscle endurance can be measured in several ways. First, the time of a sustained maximal isometric muscle contraction until 60 per cent of the initial maximal strength is left can be measured. During this test, blood supply is profoundly reduced and muscle contraction is very much dependent on anaerobic metabolism. Second, the decline in maximal force after a fixed number (18) of repetitive contractions with a fixed contraction (10 sec) and relaxation (5 sec) time can be assessed (McKenzie and Gandevia 1987). A third protocol consists of repeated contractions of 20 per cent of the maximal voluntary contractions at a pace of 12 or 30 contractions per minute up to exhaustion (Serres et al. 1998, Van 't Hul et al. 2004). This method is shown to be valid (Van 't Hul et al. 2004). The latter two are probably more related to oxidative capacity, as these dynamic muscle contractions at a low percentage of peak torque do not induce closure of capillaries in the muscle and thus do not deprive the muscle of oxygen supply.

After a specific muscle endurance training programme, significant improvements in the number of repetitions of loaded and unloaded isotonic contractions of upper and lower extremities over a 30-second period were observed (Clark et al. 1996). Although no data were shown on the reproducibility of this measurement, control subjects performed fairly reproducible results at their second visit after 12 weeks (Clark et al. 1996).

Respiratory muscle strength testing

In clinical routine, respiratory muscle strength is measured as maximal in- and expiratory mouth pressures (PImax and PEmax, respectively). These pressure measurements are made in a small cylinder attached to the mouth with a circular mouthpiece. A small leak (2 mm diameter and 15 mm length) prevents high pressures due to contraction of cheek muscles (Black and Hyatt 1969). An important part of the standardization is the lung volume from which the pressures are measured (Coast and Weise 1990). In order to prevent the contribution of chest wall and lung recoil pressure to the pressure generation of the inspiratory muscles, measurements are preferably done at FRC. However, this lung volume is difficult to standardize. In clinical practice, PImax is measured from RV whereas PEmax is taken from TLC. At least five repetitions should be performed. A recent ATS/ERS statement describes respiratory muscle testing in more detail (ATS 2002a).

Several groups developed normal values (Black and Hyatt 1969, Rochester and Arora 1983, Wilson et al. 1984) (see Table 5.5 below). Whatever normal values are used, there remains a large standard deviation. Therefore, weakness is not easy to define (Polkey et al. 1995). Inspiratory weakness is accepted when PImax is lower than 50 per cent of the predicted value (DeVito and Grassino 1995). Indeed, in studies investigating the effects of inspiratory muscle training, significant improvement in exercise performance or nocturnal desaturation time were observed in patients with a mean PImax of less than 60 per cent of the predicted value (Dekhuijzen et al. 1991, Heijdra et al. 1996, Wanke et al. 1994). Finally, respiratory muscle strength was a significant determinant of survival in patients with COPD (Decramer et al. 1996).

Table 5.5 Reference values for maximal inspiratory and expiratory mouth pressures in adults

Reference	Gender	PImax	PEmax
Black and Hyatt (1969)	M	124 ± 22	233 ± 42
	F	87 ± 16	152 ± 27
Rinqvist (1966)	M	130 ± 32	237 ± 46
	F	98 ± 25	165 ± 30
Leech et al. (1983)	M	114 ± 36	154 ± 82
	F	71 ± 27	94 ± 33
Rochester and Arora (1983)	M	127 ± 28	216 ± 41
	F	91 ± 25	138 ± 39
Wilson et al. (1984)		106 ± 31	148 ± 17
	F	73 ± 22	93 ± 17
Vincken et al. (1987)	M	105 ± 25	140 ± 38
	F	71 ± 23	89 ± 24
Bruschi et al. (1992)	M	120 ± 37	140 ± 30
	F	84 ± 30	95 ± 20

M = male   F = female

Other techniques have also been developed to assess global respiratory muscle function, such as sniff manoeuvres (Koulouris et al. 1989). The latter showed themselves to be especially reliable in testing children with neuromuscular disease. More invasive techniques such as electric or magnetic diaphragm stimulation have certainly obtained more accurate information on diaphragm function (Similowski et al. 1989, Yan et al. 1992) and are useful in the diagnosis of diaphragmatic paresis. However, for clinical application, assessment of inspiratory and expiratory mouth pressure will be sufficient.

Respiratory muscle endurance testing

Several tests for endurance capacity are described. The most frequently used are tests in which the patient breathes against a sub-maximal inspiratory load (60 to 75 per cent PImax) for as long as possible (Rochester 1988, Wanke et al. 1994). This test has been shown to be sensitive to changes after inspiratory muscle training. Incremental threshold loading, breathing against a load increased every two minutes ($\sim$5 cm H_2O), has also been shown to be reproducible (Johnson et al. 1997). The highest load that can be sustained for two minutes is the 'sustainable pressure', expressed as a percentage of the maximal load (Johnson et al. 1997, Martyn et al. 1987). Normal subjects were able to sustain 70 per cent of the PImax for two minutes (Martyn et al. 1987). Johnson et al. (1997) found that this percentage varied considerably among subjects and tended to decrease with age. The sustainable pressure has been shown to be more reduced than maximal inspiratory and expiratory pressures in COPD (van 't Hul et al. 1997). A third method (McKenzie and Gandevia 1986, McKenzie and Gandevia 1987) is repetitive maximal inspiratory or expiratory manoeuvres against an occluded airway with a well-defined contraction duration (10 sec) and relaxation time (5 sec). The relative decline in maximal pressure after 18 contractions is a measure of endurance capacity.

Tests for peripheral and respiratory muscle function are helpful in detecting muscle weakness. All these tests have their limitations, such as motivation dependency, reproducibility, availability of reference values, and costs. However, muscle weakness has been shown to be quite strongly associated with symptoms, exercise performance, utilization of health care resources, and mortality. Therefore, these measurements have become more important in clinical practice, especially when low values for muscle function are associated with clinical symptoms of weakness (fatigue, dyspnoea). The addition of tests of muscle endurance needs further research to define its contribution to the diagnosis of muscle dysfunction.

References

Agusti ACN, Barbera JA, Roca J (1990) Hypoxic pulmonary vasoconstriction and gas exchange during exercise in chronic obstructive pulmonary disease. Chest 97(2): 268–275.

Allen GM, Gandevia SC, McKenzie DK (1995) Reliability of measurements of muscle strength and voluntary activation using twitch interpolation. Muscle & Nerve 18(6): 593–600.

American Thoracic Society/European Respiratory Society (ATS) (2002a) ATS/ERS Statement on respiratory muscle testing. American Journal of Respiratory and Critical Care Medicine 166(4): 518–624.

American Thoracic Society (ATS) (2002b) ATS Statement: guidelines for the six-minute walking test. American Journal of Respiratory and Critical Care Medicine 166(4): 111–117.

Andrews AW, Thomas MW, Bohannon RW (1996) Normative values for isometric muscle force measurements obtained with hand-held dynamometers. Physical Therapy 76(3): 248–259.

Astrand I (1960) Aerobic work capacity in men and women with special reference to age. Acta Physiologica Scandinavia 49 (Supplement 169): 7–92.

Astrand PO, Saltin B (1961) Maximal oxygen uptake and heart rate in various types of muscular activity. Journal of Applied Physiology 16: 977–981.

Begin P, Grassino A (1991) Inspiratory muscle dysfunction and chronic hypercapnia in chronic obstructive pulmonary disease. American Review of Respiratory Disease 143(5 Part 1): 905–912.

Bernard S, Leblanc P, Whittom F et al. (1998) Peripheral muscle weakness in patients with chronic obstructive pulmonary disease. American Journal of Respiratory and Critical Care Medicine 158(2): 629–634.

Black LF, Hyatt RE (1969) Maximal respiratory pressures: normal values and relationship to age and sex. American Review of Respiratory Disease 99(5): 696–702.

Borges O (1989) Isometric and isokinetic knee extension and flexion torque in men and women aged 20-70. Scandinavian Journal of Rehabilitation Medicine 21(1): 45–53.

Braith RW, Graves JE, Leggett SH et al. (1993) Effect of training on the relationship between maximal and submaximal strength. Medicine and Science in Sports and Exercise 25(1): 132–138.

Bruschi C, Cerveri I, Zoia MC (1992) Reference values of maximal respiratory mouth pressures: a population-based study. American Review of Respiratory Disease 146(3): 790–793.

Casaburi R (2001) Skeletal muscle dysfunction in chronic obstructive pulmonary disease. Medicine and Science in Sports and Exercise 33(Supplement 7): S662–S700.

Casaburi R, Patessio A, Ioli F et al. (1991) Reductions in exercise lactic acidosis and ventilation as a result of exercise training in patients with obstructive lung disease. American Review of Respiratory Disease 143(1): 9–18.

Clark CJ, Cochrane JE, Mackay E (1996) Low intensity peripheral muscle conditioning improves exercise tolerance and breathlessness in COPD. European Respiratory Journal 9(12): 2590–2596.

Clark CJ, Cochrane LM, Mackay E et al. (2000) Skeletal muscle strength and endurance in patients with mild COPD and the effects of weight training. European Respiratory Journal 15(1): 92–97.

Coast JR, Weise SD (1990) Lung volume changes and maximal inspiratory pressure. Journal of Cardiopulmonary Rehabilitation 10(12): 461–464.

Cotes JE (1990) Rating respiratory disability: a report on behalf of a working group of the European Society for Clinical Respiratory Physiology. European Respiratory Journal 3(9): 1074–1077.

Debigare R, Maltais F, Mallet M et al. (2000) Influence of work rate incremental rate on the exercise responses in patients with COPD. Medicine and Science in Sports and Exercise 32(8): 1365–1368.

Decramer M, de Bock V, Dom R (1996) Functional and histologic picture of steroid-induced myopathy in chronic obstructive pulmonary disease. American Journal of Respiratory and Critical Care Medicine 153(6 Part 1): 1958–1964.

Decramer M, Demedts M, Rochette F et al. (1980) Maximal transrespiratory pressures in obstructive lung disease. Bulletin Europeen de Physiopathologie Respiratoire 16(4): 479–490.

Decramer M, Gosselink R, Troosters T et al. (1997) Muscle weakness is related to utilization of health care resources in COPD patients. European Respiratory Journal 10(2): 417–423.

Decramer M, Gosselink R, Troosters T et al. (1998) Peripheral muscle weakness is associated with reduced survival in COPD. American Journal of Respiratory and Critical Care Medicine 157: A19.

Decramer M, Lacquet LM, Fagard R et al. (1994) Corticosteroids contribute to muscle weakness in chronic airflow obstruction. American Journal of Respiratory and Critical Care Medicine 150(1): 11–16.

Dekhuijzen PN, Folgering HT, Van Herwaarden CL (1991) Target-flow inspiratory muscle training during pulmonary rehabilitation in patients with COPD. Chest 99(1): 128–133.

Dempsey JA (1986) Is the lung built for exercise? Medicine and Science in Sports and Exercise 18(2): 143–155.

DeVito E, Grassino A (1995) Respiratory muscle fatigue. Rationale for diagnostic tests. In: Roussos C (ed.) The Thorax (second edition). New York: Dekker.

Efthimiou J, Fleming J, Gomes C et al. (1988) The effect of supplementary oral nutrition in poorly nourished patients with chronic obstructive pulmonary disease. American Review of Respiratory Disease 137(5): 1075–1082.

Enright PL, Sherrill DL (1998) Reference equations for the six-minute walk in healthy adults. American Journal of Respiratory and Critical Care Medicine 158(5 Part 1): 1384–1387.

Evans AB, Al-Himyary AJ, Hrovat MI et al. (1997) Abnormal skeletal muscle oxidative capacity after lung transplantation by 31P-MRS. American Journal of Respiratory and Critical Care Medicine 155(2): 615–621.

Folgering H, Post C, Hoppenreys C (1987) Centrale en perifere exercise induced bronchoconstriction. Nederlands Tijdschrift voor Geneeskunde 131: 1646–1647.

Froelicher VF, Brammel H, Davis G et al. (1974) A comparison of the reproducibility and physiologic response to three maximal treadmill exercise protocols. Chest 65(5): 512–517.

Froelicher VF, Thompson AJ, Noguera I et al. (1975) Prediction of maximal oxygen consumption. Comparison of the Bruce and Balke protocols. Chest 68(3): 331–336.

Frontera WR, Meredith CN, O'Reilly KP et al. (1988) Strength conditioning in older men: skeletal muscle hypertrophy and improved function. Journal of Applied Physiology 64(3): 1038–1044.

Frontera WR, Meredith CN, O'Reilly KP et al. (1990) Strength training and determinants of VO$_2$ max in older men. Journal of Applied Physiology 68(1): 329–333.

Goldstein RS, Gort EH, Stubbing D et al. (1994) Randomised controlled trial of respiratory rehabilitation. Lancet 344(8934): 1394–1397.

Gosselink R, Troosters T, Decramer M (1996) Peripheral muscle weakness contributes to exercise limitation in COPD. American Journal of Respiratory and Critical Care Medicine 153(3): 976–980.

Gosselink R, Troosters T, Decramer M (2000) Distribution of respiratory and peripheral muscle weakness in patients with stable COPD. Journal of Cardiopulmonary Rehabilitation 20(6): 353–358.

Guyatt GH, Pugsley SO, Sullivan MJ et al. (1984) Effect of encouragement on walking test performance. Thorax 39(11): 818–822.

Hamilton N, Killian KJ, Summers E et al. (1995) Muscle strength, symptom intensity, and exercise capacity in patients with cardiorespiratory disorders. American Journal of Respiratory and Critical Care Medicine 152(6 Part 1): 2021–2031.

Heijdra YF, Dekhuijzen PNR, van Herwaarden CLA et al. (1996) Nocturnal saturation improves by target-flow inspiratory muscle training in patients with COPD. American Journal of Respiratory and Critical Care Medicine 153(1): 260–265.

Hermansen L, Saltin B (1969) Oxygen uptake during maximal treadmill and bicycle exercise. Journal of Applied Physiology 26(1): 31–37.

Jakobsson P, Jorfeldt L, Brundin A (1990) Skeletal muscle metabolites and fibre types in patients with advanced chronic obstructive pulmonary disease (COPD) with and without chronic respiratory failure. European Respiratory Journal 3(2): 192–196.

Johnson PH, Cowley AJ, Kinnear W (1997) Incremental threshold loading: a standard protocol and establishment of a reference range in naive normal subjects. European Respiratory Journal 10(12): 2868–2871.

Jones NL, Makrides L, Hitchcock C et al. (1985) Normal standards for an incremental progressive cycle ergometer test. American Review of Respiratory Disease 131(5): 700–708.

Kaelin ME, Swank AM, Adams KJ et al. (1999) Cardiopulmonary responses, muscle soreness, and injury during the one repetition maximum assessment in pulmonary rehabilitation patients. Journal of Cardiopulmonary Rehabilitation 19(6): 366–372.

Killian KJ, Jones NL (1988) Respiratory muscles and dyspnea. Clinics in Chest Medicine 9(2): 237–248.

Killian KJ, Leblanc P, Martin DH et al. (1992) Exercise capacity and ventilatory, circulatory, and symptom limitation in patients with chronic airflow limitation. American Review of Respiratory Disease 146(4): 935–940.

Koulouris N, Mulvey DA, Laroche CM et al. (1989) The measurement of inspiratory muscle strength by sniff esophageal, nasopharyngeal, and mouth pressures. American Review of Respiratory Disease 139(3): 641–646.

Kutsuzawa T, Shioya S, Kurita D et al. (1992) 31P-NMR study of skeletal muscle metabolism in patients with chronic respiratory impairment. American Review of Respiratory Disease 146(4): 1019–1024.

Kutsuzawa T, Shioya S, Kurita D et al. (1995) Muscle energy metabolism and nutritional status in patients with chronic obstructive pulmonary disease. A 31P magnetic resonance study. American Journal of Respiratory and Critical Care Medicine 152(2): 647–652.

Leech JA, Ghezzo H, Stevens D et al. (1983) Respiratory pressures and function in young adults. American Review of Respiratory Disease 128(1): 17–23.

Lord JP, Aitkens SG, McCrory MA et al. (1992) Isometric and isokinetic measurement of hamstring and quadriceps strength. Archives of Physical Medicine and Rehabilitation 73(4): 324–330.

Mador M, Kufel TJ, Pineda L (2000) Quadriceps fatigue after cycle exercise in patients with chronic obstructive pulmonary disease. American Journal of Respiratory and Critical Care Medicine 161(2 Part 1): 447–453.

Mak VHF, Bugler JR, Roberts CM et al. (1993) Effect of arterial oxygen desaturation on six minute walking distance, perceived effort, and perceived breathlessness in patients with airflow limitation. Thorax 48(1): 33–38.

Maltais F, Jobin J, Sullivan MJ et al. (1998) Metabolic and hemodynamic responses of lower limb during exercise in patients with COPD. Journal of Applied Physiology 84(5): 1573–1580.

Maltais F, Simard AA, Simard C et al. (1996) Oxidative capacity of the skeletal muscle and lactic acid kinetics during exercise in normal subjects and in patients with COPD. American Journal of Respiratory and Critical Care Medicine 153(1): 288–293.

Marquis K, Debigare R, Lacasse Y et al. (2002) Midthigh muscle cross-sectional area is a better predictor of mortality than body mass index in patients with chronic obstructive pulmonary disease. American Journal of Respiratory and Critical Care Medicine 166(6): 809–813.

Martyn JB, Moreno RH, Pare PD et al. (1987) Measurement of inspiratory muscle performance with incremental threshold loading. American Review of Respiratory Disease 135(4): 919–923.

Mathiowetz, V, Dove, M, Kashman N et al. (1985) Grip and pinch strength: normative data for adults. Archives of Physical Medicine and Rehabilitation 66(2): 69–72.

Mathiowetz V, Weber K, Volland G et al. (1984) Reliability and validity of grip and pinch strength evaluations. Journal of Hand Surgery 9(2): 222–226.

McArdle WD, Katch FI, Pechar GS (1973) Comparison of continuous and discontinuous treadmill and bicycle tests for max VO_2. Medicine and Science in Sports and Exercise 5(3): 156–160.

McGavin CR, Gupta SP, McHardy GJR (1976) Twelve-minute walking test for assessing disability in chronic bronchitis. British Medical Journal 1(6013): 822–823.

McKenzie DK, Gandevia SC (1986) Strength and endurance of inspiratory, expiratory and limb muscles in asthma. American Review of Respiratory Disease 134(5): 999–1004.

McKenzie DK, Gandevia SC (1987) Influence of muscle length on human inspiratory and limb muscle endurance. Respiratory Physiology 67(2): 171-182.

Merton PA (1954) Voluntary strength and fatigue. Journal of Physiology 123(3): 553-564.

Morgan AD, Peck DF, Buchanan DR et al. (1983) Effect of attitudes and beliefs on exercise tolerance in chronic bronchitis. British Medical Journal 286(6360): 171–173.

Neder JA, Jones PW, Nery LE et al. (2000) Determinants of exercise endurance capacity in patients with chronic obstructive pulmonary disease. The power–duration relationship. American Journal of Respiratory and Critical Care Medicine 162(2 Part 1): 497–504.

Neder JA, Nery LE, Shinzato GT et al. (1999) Reference values for concentric knee isokinetic strength and power in non-athletic men and women from 20 to 80 years old. Journal of Orthopaedic and Sports Physical Therapy 29(2): 116–126.

Newell SZ, McKenzie DK, Gandevia SC (1989) Inspiratory and skeletal muscle strength and endurance and diaphragmatic activation in patients with chronic airflow limitation. Thorax 44(11): 903–912.

O'Donnell DE (2002) Exercise limitation and clinical exercise testing in chronic obstructive pulmonary disease. In: Idelle M, Weisman R, Jorge Z (eds.) Clinical Exercise Testing. Basel: Karger.

O'Donnell DE, McGuire MA, Samis L et al. (1998) General exercise training improves ventilatory and peripheral muscle strength and endurance in chronic airflow limitation. American Journal of Respiratory and Critical Care Medicine 157(5 Part 1): 1489–1497.

O'Donnell DE, Webb KA (1998) Measurement of symptoms, lung hyperinflation, and endurance during exercise in chronic obstructive pulmonary disease. American Journal of Respiratory and Critical Care Medicine 158(5 Part 1): 1557–1565.

Palange P, Galassetti P, Mannix ET et al. (1995) Oxygen effect on O_2 deficit and VO_2 kinetics during exercise in obstructive pulmonary disease. Journal of Applied Physiology 78(6): 2228–2234.

Pardy RL, Rivington RN, Despas PJ et al. (1981) The effects of inspiratory muscle training on exercise performance in chronic airflow limitation. American Review of Respiratory Disease 123(4 Part 1): 426–433.

Payen J-P, Wuyam B, Levy P et al. (1993) Muscular metabolism during oxygen supplementation in patients with chronic hypoxemia. American Review of Respiratory Disease 147(3): 592–598.

Perez T, Becquart LA, Stach B et al. (1996) Inspiratory muscle strength and endurance in steroid-dependent asthma. American Journal of Respiratory and Critical Care Medicine 153(2): 610–615.

Phillips BA, Lo SK, Mastaglia FL (2000) Muscle force measured using 'break' testing with a hand-held myometer in normal subjects aged 20 to 69 years. Archives of Physical Medicine and Rehabilitation 81(5): 653–661.

Polkey MI, Green M, Moxham J (1995) Measurement of respiratory muscle strength. Thorax 50(11): 1131–1135.

Polkey MI, Kyroussis D, Harris ML et al. (1996) Are voluntary manoeuvres maximal in routine clinical testing? American Journal of Respiratory and Critical Care Medicine 153: A785.

Redelmeier DA, Bayoumi AM, Goldstein RS et al. (1997) Interpreting small differences in functional status: the six-minute walk test in chronic lung disease patients. American Journal of Respiratory and Critical Care Medicine 155(4): 1278–1282.

Revill SM, Morgan MDL, Singh SJ et al. (1999) The endurance shuttle walk: a new field test for the assessment of endurance capacity in chronic obstructive pulmonary disease. Thorax 54(3): 213–222.

Rinqvist T (1966) The ventilatory capacity in healthy adults: an analysis of causal factors with special reference to the respiratory forces. Scandinavian Journal of Clinical Laboratory Investigation 88: 5–179 (Supplement).

Rochester D, Arora NS (1983) Respiratory muscle failure. Medical Clinics of North America 67(3): 573–598.

Rochester DF (1988) Tests of respiratory muscle function. Clinics in Chest Medicine 9(2): 249–261.

Rochester DF, Braun NMT (1985) Determinants of maximal inspiratory pressure in chronic obstructive pulmonary disease. American Review of Respiratory Disease 132(1): 42–47.

Serres I, Gautier V, Varray A et al. (1998) Impaired skeletal muscle endurance related to physical inactivity and altered lung function in COPD patients. Chest 113(4): 900–905.

Similowski T, Fleury B, Launois S et al. (1989) Cervical magnetic stimulation: a new painless method for bilateral phrenic nerve stimulation in conscious humans. Journal of Applied Physiology 67(4): 1311–1318.

Simpson K, Killian KJ, McCartney N et al. (1992) Randomised controlled trial of weightlifting exercise in patients with chronic airflow limitation. Thorax 47(2): 70–75.

Singh SJ, Morgan MDL, Hardman AE et al. (1994) Comparison of oxygen uptake during conventional treadmill test and the shuttle walking test in chronic airflow limitation. European Respiratory Journal 7(11): 2016–2020.

Singh SJ, Morgan MDL, Scott S et al. (1992) The development of the shuttle walking test of disability in patients with chronic airways obstruction. Thorax 47(12): 1019–1024.

Solway S, Brooks D, Lacasse Y et al. (2001) A qualitative systematic overview of the measurement properties of functional walk tests used in the cardiorespiratory domain. Chest 119(1): 256–270.

Stevens D, Elpern E, Sharma K et al. (1999) Comparison of hallway and treadmill six-minute walk tests. American Journal of Respiratory and Critical Care Medicine 160(5 Part 1): 1540–1543.

Stratford PW, Balsor BE (1994) A comparison of make and break tests using a hand-held dynamometer and the Kin-Com. Journal of Orthopaedic and Sports Physical Therapy 19(1): 28–32.

Swinburn CR, Wakefield JM, Jones PW (1985) Performance, ventilation, and oxygen consumption in three different types of exercise test in patients with chronic obstructive lung disease. Thorax 40(8): 581–586.

Troosters T, Gosselink R, Decramer M (1999a) Reliability of handheld myometry to measure peripheral muscle strength in COPD. European Respiratory Journal 14: 481.

Troosters T, Gosselink R, Decramer M (1999b) Six-minute walking distance in healthy elderly subjects. European Respiratory Journal 14(2): 270-274.

Troosters T, Gosselink R, Decramer M (2000a) How accurate are measures of peripheral muscle with hand held myometry? American Journal of Respiratory and Critical Care Medicine 161: A752.

Troosters T, Gosselink R, Decramer M (2000b) Short- and long-term effects of outpatient pulmonary rehabilitation in COPD patients: a randomized controlled trial. American Journal of Medicine 109(3): 207–212.

Troosters T, Gosselink R, Decramer M (2001) Exercise training in COPD: how to distinguish responders from non-responders. Journal of Cardiopulmonary Rehabilitation 21(1): 10–17.

Troosters T, Gosselink R, Rollier H et al. (1996a) Change in lower limb muscle strength contributes to altered six minute walking distance in COPD. European Respiratory Journal 9 A752.

Troosters T, Gosselink R, Rollier H et al. (1996b) Increases in peripheral muscle strength contribute to improved quality of life in COPD patients. American Journal of Respiratory and Critical Care Medicine 153: A425.

Troosters T, Vilaro J, Rabinovich R et al. (2002) Physiological responses to the six-minute walk test in patients with chronic obstructive pulmonary disease. European Respiratory Journal 20(3): 564–569.

van der Ploeg RJO, Fidler V, Oosterhuis JHGH (1991) Hand-held myometry: reference values. Journal of Neurology, Neurosurgery, and Psychiatry 54(3): 244–247.

van Stel HF, Bogaard JM, Rijssenbeek-Nouwens LH et al. (2001) Multivariable assessment of the six-minute walking test in patients with chronic obstructive pulmonary disease. American Journal of Respiratory and Critical Care Medicine 163(7): 1567–1571.

van 't Hul AJ, Chadwick-Straver RVM, Wagenaar RC et al. (1997) Inspiratory muscle endurance is reduced more than maximal respiratory pressures in COPD patients. European Respiratory Journal 10: 168S.

van 't Hul AJ, Gosselink R, Kwakkel G (2003) Constant-load cycle endurance performance: test–retest reliability and validity in patients with COPD. Journal of Cardiopulmonary Rehabilitation 23(2): 143–150.

van 't Hul AJ, Harlaar J, Gosselink R, Hollander P, Postmus P, Kwakkel G (2004) Quadriceps muscle endurance in patients with chronic obstructive pulmonary disease. Muscle Nerve 29(1): 267–279.

Vincken W, Ghezzo H, Cosio MG (1987) Maximal static respiratory pressures in adults: normal values and their relationship to determinants of respiratory function. Bulletin Europeen de Physiopathologie Respiratoire 23(5): 435–439.

Wanke T, Formanek D, Lahrmann H et al. (1994) The effects of combined inspiratory muscle and cycle ergometer training on exercise performance in patients with COPD. European Respiratory Journal 7(12): 2205–2211.

Wasserman K, Hansen JE, Sue DY et al. (1994) Principles of Exercise Testing and Interpretation (second edition). Philadelphia, Pa: Lea & Febiger.

Wasserman K, Sue DY, Casaburi R et al. (1989) Selection criteria for exercise training in pulmonary rehabilitation. European Respiratory Journal 7: 604S–610S.

Weisman R, Jorge Z (eds.) (2002) Clinical Exercise Testing. Basel: Karger.

Whipp BJ, Wagner PD, Agusti A (1998) Factors determining the response to exercise in healthy subjects. In: Roca J, Whipp BJ (eds.) Clinical Exercise Testing 2(6): 3–31.

Whittom F, Jobin J, Simard P-M et al. (1998) Histochemical and morphological characteristics of the vastus lateralis muscle in patients with chronic obstructive pulmonary disease. Medicine and Science in Sports and Exercise 30(10): 1467–1474.

Wijkstra PJ, Ten Vergert EM, Van der Mark TW et al. (1994) Relation of lung function, maximal inspiratory pressure, dyspnoea, and quality of life with exercise capacity in patients with chronic obstructive pulmonary disease. Thorax 49(5): 468–472.

Wilson DO, Cooke NT, Edwards RHT et al. (1984) Predicted normal values for maximal respiratory pressures in Caucasian adults and children. Thorax 39(7): 535–538.

Wilson DO, Rogers RM, Sanders MH et al. (1986) Nutritional intervention in malnourished patients with emphysema. American Review of Respiratory Disease 134(4): 672–677.

Wilson GJ, Murphy AJ (1996) Strength diagnosis: the use of test data to determine specific strength training. Journal of Sports Sciences 14(2): 167–173.

Wilson RC, Jones PW (1991) Differentiation between the intensity of breathlessness and the distress it evokes in normal subjects during exercise. Clinical Science 80(1): 65–70.

Yan S, Gauthier AP, Similowski T et al. (1992) Evaluation of human contractility using mouth pressure twitches. American Review of Respiratory Disease 145(5): 1064–1069.

Zattara-Hartmann MC, Badier M, Guillot C et al. (1995) Maximal force and endurance to fatigue of respiratory and skeletal muscles in chronic hypoxemic patients: the effects of oxygen breathing. Muscle & Nerve 18(5): 495–502.

Chapter 6
COPD: a biopsychosocial approach

M. FITZPATRICK, J. FEARN

Introduction

Chronic obstructive pulmonary disease (COPD) is an umbrella term that encompasses emphysema, chronic bronchitis and irreversible asthma (Toshima et al. 1992). Patients with COPD exhibit features of each of these in varying degrees, and the main characteristic is dyspnoea with a number of physical sequelae (Tregonning and Langley 1999). Although there are a number of potential contributory factors to the development and onset of COPD, smoking is the main cause. Doll et al. (1994) indicate that smoking is accountable for 80 per cent of the attributable risk. Unsurprisingly, smoking cessation is the single most effective way of altering outcome in this patient group, although COPD itself is irreversible (Halpin 2001).

COPD, like other chronic conditions, may be usefully framed within a biopsychosocial model (Engel 1977). This emphasizes the link between the body and the mind. It is a framework within which the biological, psychological and social aspects of physical conditions may be integrated. The biopsychosocial model helps to explain the processes involved in chronic physical conditions such as COPD (Figure 6.1). It sets a meaningful agenda for patients with a physical condition that affects mobility, functional activity, mood/affect and aspects within the social context and family systems. The biopsychosocial approach promotes a sense of self-efficacy not only for the patient but also for the health care professional.

Self-efficacy refers to a person's belief that they can perform or engage in a particular activity or achieve a designated task or goal. In patients with COPD, self-efficacy expectation is related to dyspnoea. These beliefs influence how much people do, what course of action they take, how much effort they put in, and how long they persevere (Bandura 1992a, 1992b, 1997, Krall et al. 1997). The emphasis of intervention is management rather than the absence of cure. This is reflected in recent guidelines that emphasize the need for pulmonary rehabilitation of COPD patients to improve aspects such as quality of life, independence

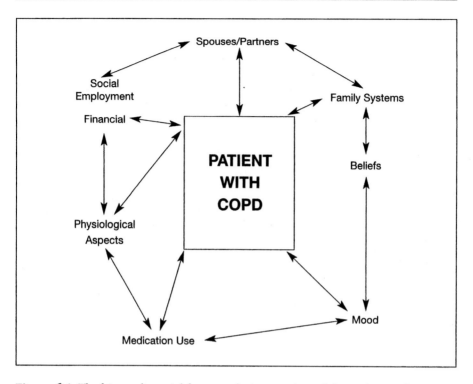

Figure 6.1 The biopsychosocial framework. An overview of the patient with COPD.

and psychological well-being. (BTS 1997, ATS 1995). Finally, a biopsy-chosocial approach to the management of COPD lends itself to multidisciplinary working.

Patients with COPD are likely to be in the older adult age group (Yohannes et al. 2000). Many patients with mild disease are not diagnosed and do not consult their doctors. Therefore, by inference, a number of years may have elapsed between disease onset and diagnosis. By this stage, symptoms already make a significant impact upon patients' quality of life (Halpin 2001). They describe significant difficulties in maintaining normal levels of activity, loss of fitness and mobility and increased levels of fatigue (Yohannes et al. 2000). They may, as a result of functional limi-tations, have gained or lost weight and may describe disrupted sleep. As symptoms continue to worsen, patients may also report mood changes, such as frustration, anger, low mood and anxiety. These feelings may be related to an inability to complete everyday tasks, the unpredictability of the symptoms experienced, or the degree to which the disease process dominates day-to-day life. Breathlessness, the main physical characteristic of the condition, may provoke feelings of anxiety. Patients may express fears about the future and the likelihood of deterioration. Such fears may induce panic responses to breathlessness and an overriding fear of respiratory failure (Schrier et al. 1990, McSweeney and Labuhn 1990).

Patients of working age may find it difficult to maintain employment, and take early or medical retirement. This may result in a change of roles both within and without the home. Other knock-on effects include difficulties maintaining a sexual relationship, social life, hobbies and interests (Hanson 1982). Breathlessness following increased exertion and loss of fitness maintains these difficulties. So does anxiety. It is a by-product, at least in part, of the deconditioning process. Quality of life in each of these aspects is therefore likely to be seriously impaired (Yohannes et al. 2000).

Most people with COPD will use inhalers and/or nebulizers as a long-term way of controlling and stabilizing symptoms. Some drugs have the effect of opening up the airways to relieve symptoms of breathlessness, while others containing small amounts of steroids have the effect of dampening down inflammation. Inhalers and nebulizers are aimed at controlling physical symptoms and are not curative. Medication, however, does not always provide relief from symptoms. With long-term use, patients often describe negative side effects, such as shaking and palpitations, oral thrush or thinning of the outer layers of the skin leading to easy bruising.

COPD and depression

There is some degree of variability across studies about the prevalence of depression in COPD patients. In a meta-analysis of nine studies, Yohannes et al. (2000) estimate the prevalence of depression in patients with COPD to be 40 per cent with a range of 36 to 44 per cent. Van Manen et al. (2002) examined the issue of severity of COPD and depression. Outcomes from this control study suggest that 21.6 per cent of the COPD population suffer/experience depression. They divided patients into mild to moderate and severe groups. The mild to moderate COPD group had a depression prevalence of 19.6 per cent; the severe group had a depression prevalence of 25 per cent, and controls a depression prevalence of 17.5 per cent.

Results were adjusted for confounding variables, including demographics, and they addressed the important issue of co-morbidity. In the multivariate analysis there appeared to be no risk for depression in the total group of COPD patients, or in the subgroup of patients with mild to moderate COPD. Conversely, those who had severe COPD had a 2.5 times greater risk for depression than controls.

Van Manen et al.'s 2002 study highlights an increased risk for depression for those living alone, patients with reversibility in FEV_1 (forced expiratory volume in one second) of less than or equal to 1.1 per cent and those with COPD with severe impaired physical functioning. They comment that prevalence rates of depression for COPD patients in previous studies ranged from 6 to 46 per cent. They question how this was measured and suggest that methodological issues may account for the degree of variability reported. The conclusion drawn is that the perceived severity of the disease seems to be at least as important as the clinically assessed severity for developing depression. Focusing on decreasing symptoms and improving functioning by rehabilitation programmes and by psychosocial intervention may, they conclude, decrease depression rates.

COPD and anxiety

Yohannes et al. (2000) estimate the prevalence of anxiety in COPD patients to be 36 per cent with a range of 31 to 41 per cent. In a study which took a cognitive-behavioural focus and looked specifically at the role of thoughts, Sutton et al. (1999) report that severe catastrophic thoughts are associated with increased levels of anxiety in patients with COPD. They also state that this is more important than the duration or severity of the condition itself.

An approach to assessment

Sending patients an information leaflet about the assessment process and possible interventions will help them make a decision about whether to attend or not. It is vital that patient leaflets are user-friendly. Individual trusts are likely to provide guidelines and quality assessors to help ensure this. Attention is drawn to the Flesch Formula, which is a technique of assessing readability of patient leaflets (Flesch 1948).

Patients are assessed with a view to intervention. This may be on a one-to-one or a group basis. A cognitive-behavioural approach, which will be outlined here, is consonant with a biopsychosocial perspective. It underlines the links between thoughts, feelings, behaviours, physiological components and the social context. This reflects the key components of the cognitive-behavioural model of rehabilitation, which comprises education, skills training, cognitive intervention, behavioural goals, exercise, relaxation, and spouse/carers involvement.

For group rehabilitation programmes it is recommended that multidisciplinary collaboration starts at assessment. Staff may include a respiratory nurse specialist, a physiotherapist and a clinical psychologist. The assessment process should take place within a set of clearly established inclusion and exclusion criteria. These may include:

- Is the person motivated/do they want to take part in an intervention aimed at managing their condition either on a one-to-one or at group level?
- What changes do they want to make?
- Can they commit to attendance and participation?
- Is their mood sufficient to engage (is the patient too depressed, for example, to take on board the challenges of working in a group)?

- Are there other concurrent issues that may militate against successful participation (for example alcohol dependency)?
- Can the person read and write?
- Are there concurrent psychiatric conditions for which they are receiving/should receive psychiatric intervention and which are paramount?
- Are there practical issues about access to the venue?
- Is the person a smoker? Some multidisciplinary staff groups may exclude smokers. A prerequisite to group intervention may be successful completion of a smoking-cessation intervention.

It is useful to invite a spouse, carer or partner to assessment. This is important for a number of reasons. It may elucidate the extent to which they are positively/negatively reinforcing passive or active management strategies. This may be assessed by asking questions such as:

- 'How do you respond when your partner is having a bad day?'
- 'Do you often suggest that your partner rests?'
- 'What are your feelings about your partner exercising or walking?'

The inclusion of the spouse may elucidate the degree to which they may be over-involved or under-involved in supporting their partner/spouse. What they say can provide useful information about how their partner has changed over time, for example with regard to mobility, activity and mood. It is also an opportunity for each of the health care professionals to begin to address carers' anxieties about their relatives and to begin the process of educating them. Data indicate, for example, that the well-being of wives with COPD partners is reduced because of the care-giving tasks they undertake (Cossette and Levesque 1993).

Assessment should cover the following areas:

Assessment components

Preparation
- read medical/psychiatric notes

Assessment interview
- history of COPD and symptomatology
- duration of chest problem
- perceived progression
- understanding of condition (knowledge base)
- beliefs about condition
- exacerbating and moderating factors

Medical interventions
- past and current treatment
- what has/has not helped?
- understanding of medication and adherence
- frequency of medication use and side effects
- any other past or concurrent medical history?

Impact of COPD on:
- family
- social life
- employment
- activities of daily living

Coping strategies
- identification of current management strategies
- passive
- active
- avoidant

Assessment of mood
- symptoms of depression and anxiety
- psychological/psychiatric history
- current psychological/psychiatric input

Motivation to change
- expectations of intervention
- identification of goals/desired changes

What the spouse/relative has to say
- how does COPD affect them?
- what thoughts/beliefs do they have about COPD?
- responses to the person with COPD.

Measures

There are a number of issues in relation to the use of questionnaires. These include 'What do we measure?', 'How do we measure it?' and 'What relevance does this have to the outcomes we are looking for?' There are a number of established generic questionnaires available, but a dearth of COPD-specific scales. Established generic questionnaires include the Hospital Anxiety and Depression (HAD) scale (Snaith and Zigmond 1994), which is designed to detect symptoms of anxiety and depression. It is a 14-item self-report questionnaire that is quick and easy to administer. It avoids some of the physiological items found in other scales and was originally intended for use with non-psychiatric hospital departments. It does not rely on symptoms that might be present in people with physical illness alone. The HAD does not set out to be a diagnostic measure, but it is a useful way of monitoring change in symptoms over time (Zigmond and Snaith 1983).

A widely used measure of health status is the SF36 (Ware et al. 1993). It is a multi-item scale that assesses physical functioning, role limitations, social functioning, bodily pain, general mental health, vitality and general health perception. It has been shown to measure and quantify changes in quality of life functions. It has good reliability and validity.

The St George's Respiratory Questionnaire (SGRQ) is a COPD-specific self-report measure that sets out to identify patients' perceptions of their health-related quality of life. The questionnaire has 76 items covering symptoms, activity, and the impact of COPD (Jones et al. 1992). The questionnaire has a complex scoring system, but has been found to have good test–retest reliability and validity (Randall Curtis et al. 1996).

The COPD self-efficacy questionnaire (Wigal et al. 1991) comprises 34 items and has proven good test–retest reliability, according to the authors. Reliability is limited, however, because the scale reliability was established with a small self-selected number of participants. The authors do not comment upon any aspect of validity.

A cognitive-behavioural programme

The following approaches provide examples of how behaviour and cognitions can interact with physiological changes to cause feelings of depression and anxiety. Individual assessment of patients requires detailed discussion of cognitions and beliefs affecting behaviour. In this way therapists can assist patients in combating false beliefs which may be affecting their mood state and behaviour.

Pacing

A common behaviour pattern of patients with COPD (and other chronic conditions) is the overactivity/underactivity cycle (Figure 6.2). This can be explained by the patient's need to fight their condition and attempts to maintain normal levels of activity at all costs. Too much activity can lead to an increased frequency or severity of symptoms and enforced rest periods often lasting for days. This further affects mood and decreases self-efficacy. Over time, this pattern may become established and may lead to decreases in levels of activity, deconditioning and fear avoidance.

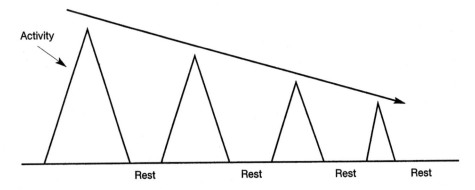

Figure 6.2 Overactivity/underactivity cycle.

One way of breaking into the overactivity/underactivity cycle is pacing. Pacing essentially describes a way of breaking activities down into small, easily achievable parts. Activities will inevitably take longer using this process; however, it means that patients experience the satisfaction and achievement of completing a task without exacerbating their symptoms. Pacing results in enhanced self-efficacy and improved mood. It helps patients to remain physically active.

A paced approach to activity and exercise produces a controllable level of breathlessness (Figure 6.3). This, alongside education/information about breathlessness and activity, helps to alter patients' beliefs about it. This increases their sense of control, reduces anxiety, and they experience a sense of achievement.

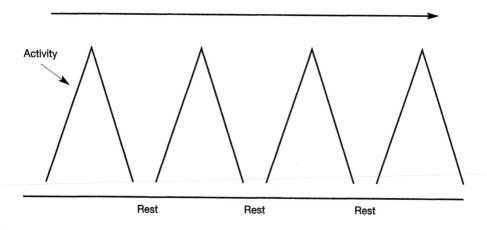

Figure 6.3 A paced approach to activity.

Characteristically, people have a number of cognitive barriers to pacing. These may include, for example:

- 'In the past I used to be able to do this without thinking twice.'
- 'It's either all or nothing with me.'
- 'I've got to get this done today.'
- 'I should be able to do this.'
- 'There's no point walking. I get short of breath really easily.'

These cognitions can be challenged by both behaviour change and its positive outcomes and by use of cognitive strategies, to be discussed later.

Pacing: setting a baseline

This can be applied to most activities. It involves targeting activities of daily living and recording how long patients can comfortably continue with these before breathlessness prevents them continuing. These recordings are completed (using a timer) over the course of several days to produce a realistic picture of an activity across good and bad days. Recordings are then averaged and reduced by 20 per cent to provide a realistic baseline, which the patient can adhere to on good and bad days. Once this has been set, patients are asked to maintain this level for a specific period of time. This continues until they can routinely engage in the activity without negative consequences, such as pushing themselves into distress and extreme breathlessness. The baseline is then increased over time in a planned way. It helps to improve fitness and activity levels.

Goal-setting

Goals have an important function in life. They provide a sense of pleasure and/or achievement. Many patients with COPD have stopped or reduced these activities because of breathlessness or a fear of breathlessness.

SMART

A key way of helping patients identify goals is to ask them to think about activities they have stopped as a result of COPD. Goals need to be self-selected to be meaningful and to motivate patients to engage with their own treatment. Alongside these, staff will also negotiate other goals, for example a 30-minute walk five times a week, or a relaxation session once a day three times a week. Thus goals are a product of patient/therapist negotiation. Once goals have been identified it can be difficult to know how to get started. A common approach can be summarized in the acronym SMART. This means that goals are:

Specific: The more specific a goal, the easier it is to identify when it has been achieved. Specific examples are: 'I shall prune the roses twice a week', 'I shall take a regular walk once a day', 'I shall practise relaxation daily', rather than non-specific examples such as: 'I want to be able to do more gardening', 'I want to get fit', 'I want to become less anxious'.

Measurable: Goals may be measured either by frequency, in time, or both. Example: 'I shall walk five times a week for ten minutes', 'I shall practise relaxation for 30 minutes three times a week'.

Achievable and **R**ealistic: The key to making goals achievable is to use the baseline process described earlier. Common sense and clear judgement need to be used. For most people, running a marathon may not be achievable or realistic. There may also be financial or social constraints, and those imposed by other physical and medical conditions.

Time Bound: This means setting a starting date, deciding frequency and duration, and setting a date for review. Patients are asked to make a contract with themselves to attempt the goal within a planned time-frame.

Rewards

The final step in goal-setting involves the identification of a suitable reward. Rewards motivate and reinforce the recognition that a goal has been achieved. Rewards need to be changed over time otherwise they lose their effectiveness.

How to help COPD patients manage depression and anxiety symptoms

A cognitive-behavioural approach to managing anxiety and depression includes helping patients to identify catastrophic or negative automatic thinking. This helps patients understand how thoughts affect feelings, physiological sensations, what they do and/or what they avoid (Figure 6.4).

There are some features common to depressed mood and COPD and anxiety and COPD (Figures 6.4 and 6.5). These include, for example, decreased physical activity, breathlessness, sleep disruption and loss of appetite. Education about depression and anxiety can help target symptoms more appropriately. Patients also learn to attribute physical symptoms more appropriately.

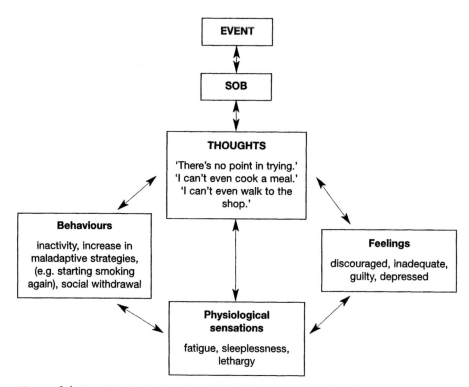

Figure 6.4 Cognitive-behavioural model of depressed mood and COPD.

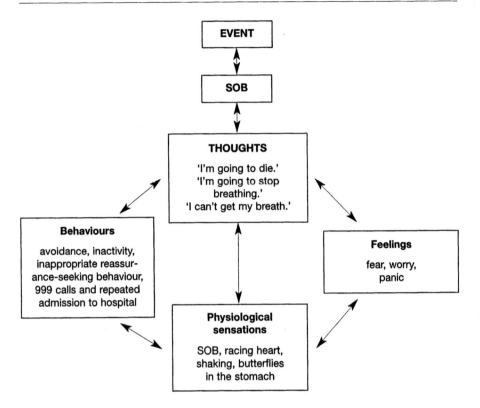

Figure 6.5 Cognitive-behavioural model of anxiety and COPD.

Using a cognitive-behavioural framework involves the identification of negative automatic thoughts (NATs) and recognition of how these influence emotions, physiological sensations and behaviour.

NATs (negative automatic thoughts)

- pop into your head
- are involuntary
- do not fit all the facts
- affect how you feel
- affect what you do
- affect what you avoid
- affect how your body reacts.

Patients with COPD often have, for example, catastrophizing thoughts, which increase the likelihood of feelings of fear, worry and apprehension. This fear generates further somatic symptoms of anxiety, including hyperventilation. Together, these can increase the likelihood of avoidance behaviours. This may result in inappropriate reassurance-seeking behaviours such as frequent GP visits, 999 calls, overuse of medication and presentation at A & E departments (Salkovskis et al. 1986).

Patients are encouraged to learn how to challenge their catastrophic or negative automatic thoughts by the use of strategies such as looking at the evidence for their beliefs and by identifying more rational and balanced responses.

Challenging NATs

Three key questions:

1. What is the evidence for the thought?
2. What are the consequences of leaving these thoughts unchallenged?
3. Is there another way of thinking about this?

Types of thinking mistakes

Patients are taught how to identify their NATs, and common examples include:

Catastrophizing: Catastrophic thoughts might include the belief that breathlessness is always an indication of further damage to the lungs or that respiratory failure is imminent. Catastrophizing thoughts are about envisaging the worst-case scenario.

Generalization: This is the belief that breathlessness, in one situation, will inevitably occur in all similar situations, for example a person might experience an episode of breathlessness in a supermarket and believe this will always occur on subsequent visits to the supermarket.

All or nothing thinking: This way of thinking can lead patients to give up certain activities completely because they can no longer complete them as before.

Mind reading: This is when people assume that they know what others are thinking. These are usually negative in content, and people tend to respond to what they think someone is thinking rather than checking it out or challenging it.

Cognitive diaries

Asking patients to keep cognitive diaries is part of the process of learning how to recognize and challenge NATs. It involves asking patients to monitor how they are feeling and to recall so-called negative-affect or physiological sensations, for example breathlessness, pain or low mood. Patients are encouraged to focus on what situation they are in or what they are thinking about generally. This helps them identify specific NATs. They are then asked to write down rational responses to these NATs by using the information they have been given about types of thinking errors and how to challenge them. Having done this, patients then review how they feel and their physiological sensations and note outcomes. This is likely to result in reduced anxiety, depression and/or breathlessness as a result of challenging the thoughts and using coping strategies, such as relaxation and distraction.

Biofeedback

A helpful adjunct to the management of anxiety is the use of biofeedback. This can take the form of, for example, pulse recordings, measures of electrodermal activity or oxygen saturation levels, and is usually recorded before and after exercise. Feeding back the pulse rate to the patient following exercise, and seeing it drop back to normal can reinforce that breathlessness need not be dangerous. It may also help to challenge catastrophizing thoughts. Biofeedback can also help to identify when patients overexert themselves, and underlines the need to pace or adjust the level of activity.

Relaxation

Relaxation, either on a one-to-one basis or in a group setting, is a useful technique. It promotes a sense of self-efficacy in the management of breathlessness and the psychological and somatic components of anxiety. Explaining the necessity of practice to master the skill of relaxation is important, and there are a variety of techniques that may be used. These include autogenic, progressive muscular, visualization, or a combination of these and others (Jacobson 1929).

The opportunity for practice with the health care professional is important. Provision of a tape recording of relaxation exercises may enhance adherence. Care needs to be taken when using relaxation, as it may adversely affect some physical conditions, for example the lowering of blood-sugar levels in people with insulin-dependent diabetes.

Education/information giving

Education and information giving may, in themselves, reduce anxiety and increase adherence. Sessions with a particular focus on education may include:

- what is COPD? (delivered by a thoracic respiratory physician or nurse specialist)
- the benefits of exercise
- understanding medications, i.e. inhalers, nebulizers, oxygen therapy
- when to go to your GP
- balanced, healthy eating
- benefits information (practical information that may lead to decreased financial stresses)
- going on holiday.

Spouse/carer's involvement

In a group intervention, it is useful to invite spouses/carers to the information-giving/education session provided by the respiratory physician or nurse. A shared understanding of the condition helps to reduce anxiety and redress under- or over-involvement of the spouse or carer. For those patients involved in an individual intervention, the spouse or carer can be invited to a three-way session with the clinical psychologist, or they may be referred to a clinical nurse specialist for input. Giving spouses/carers opportunities to meet with other spouses/carers also reduces their anxiety and helps them find more appropriate ways of supporting their spouse/partner as they seek ways of managing their condition. Together, they can also plan joint goals for the future.

Working with individuals and groups

The group experience offers patients an opportunity to observe how other members of the group make changes. It gives an opportunity for behaviour modelling. A number of elements contribute to the dynamics of a group.

Relevance

Not all sessions will be equally relevant to those working in a group context. It is important that people understand why these topics feature in the programme and that these may be especially important to other members of the group. Clinicians should include and encourage participation by everyone.

Ground rules

It is useful during the introductory session to set ground rules. These need to appear relevant for patients and be understood as a way of facilitating the rehabilitative process.

Working with challenging patients

Working with challenging patients is important. They may disrupt the therapeutic progress and can leave others feeling frightened, anxious or angry. While group members are encouraged to take responsibility for the group, ultimately it is the responsibility of clinicians to maximize a positive outcome. Therefore, this may necessitate discussion with the individual during the group process, or outside of the group, in order to come to an understanding of the factors precipitating challenging behaviour. These exchanges should be about problem resolution rather than being punitive in nature. Occasional use of 'time-out' during a programme may sometimes benefit the individual and the group.

Time-out in this context simply means that patients refrain from verbal interactions for the duration of that part of the session.

Working with silent patients

Reinforcing any verbal contributions from participants who are normally quiet helps to encourage more interaction. Encouraging responses and contributions from every member of the group on a particular issue or question gives the opportunity in a non-threatening way for the silent person to contribute. It is important to find out the underlying reason for a participant's silence. Do not assume that the underlying cause is anxiety or disengagement.

Non-attendance

Patients do not attend for a variety of reasons. These might include anxiety or difficulty engaging with the group. It is important to find out why non-attendance occurs. Patients who do not attend should be reminded of the ground rules set out at the introductory session. These include the importance of attending all sessions unless a significant exacerbation of their condition occurs, or some other unexpected significant event. Attendance underlines commitment to the group.

Homework tasks

It is important that patients understand that homework tasks are an integral part of the programme. Any completion of homework should be reinforced to encourage further work. Having been set, it is essential that homework tasks are followed up. Homework tasks may include cognitive diaries, monitoring goals, completing exercise sheets or practising relaxation.

Maintenance and relapse prevention

While one of the major aims of a cognitive-behavioural intervention with COPD patients is to promote self-efficacy, follow-up at, for example, three, six and 12 months gives opportunities to address maintenance and relapse issues. Patients will have a copy of an action plan that they can use, for example after hospitalization or a relapse due to other circumstances. An action plan may include:

- get back to monitoring
- reset baselines for exercise
- call another member of the group
- re-read handouts given during the programme
- write down goals achieved so far
- use a cognitive diary

- call a staff member to discuss getting started again.

Follow-up sessions also provide longer-term clinical outcomes via, for example, self-report and questionnaires, recordings of number of hospitalizations, and recompleting walking assessments.

Smoking cessation

No chapter on the psychosocial aspects of COPD would be complete without a discussion about smoking cessation. It has been clearly demonstrated that smoking cessation is the single most important thing a person with COPD can do. It is essential, therefore, to offer intervention to meet this goal. Smoking cessation may be offered on a one-to-one or group basis. It may be part of a wider group intervention for people with COPD, or it may be a prerequisite to participating in a group rehabilitation programme.

It is important that the smoker is motivated to stop. This can be encouraged or fostered by helping the patient to understand the reasons behind the smoking behaviour and the balance between the short-term and long-term advantages and disadvantages of continuing or stopping. Reinforcing the smoker's identified reasons for stopping is important. Enhancing self-efficacy is also crucial.

Appropriate behavioural modifications need to replace the reward of smoking. Patients need specific techniques to help with the psychological and pharmacological aspects of what appears an impossible task. It is beyond the scope of this chapter to review and present smoking-cessation interventions, but there is an expansive literature on the subject. Readers are encouraged to examine some of the social cognition theories, the health belief model, the theory of planned behaviour, and Prochaska and Diclemente's stages of change model (Prochaska and Diclemente 1983, Prochaska et al. 1992). This latter transtheoretical model of change aims to offer a general, theoretical and coherent account of behaviour change. Interestingly, more recent applications of the model have been to smoking cessation. The model postulates five stages of change:

1. **precontemplation** or not seriously thinking about change
2. **contemplation** or seriously thinking about change
3. **preparation** or a readiness to change
4. **action** or attempting to change
5. **maintenance** or change achieved.

The model suggests that people move through these stages in a dynamic, rather than a linear, fashion. A person might, for example, move from preparation to action and back several times before moving on to the maintenance stage. Prochaska and Diclemente called this process 'the revolving door' schema. This suggests that, even if change has not been maintained, there is a process of learning. The model also suggests that it is possible to reach the maintenance stage and then relapse back into pre-contemplation (Ogden 1996).

Summary

This chapter outlines a biopsychosocial approach to the management of patients with COPD. It describes the constituent components of a cognitive-behavioural intervention, with particular emphasis on multidisciplinary group working. It highlights relevant literature that will give the reader an understanding of both the theoretical underpinnings and clinical applications.

References

ATS (1995) Standards for the diagnosis and care of patients with chronic obstructive pulmonary disease. American Thoracic Society. American Journal of Respiratory and Critical Care Medicine 152(5 Part 2): S77–S121.

Bandura A (1992a) Exercise of personal agency through the self-efficacy mechanism. In: Schwarzer R (ed.) Self-efficacy: Thought Control of Action. Washington DC: Hemisphere Publishing.

Bandura A (1992b) Self-efficacy mechanism in psychobiologic functioning. In: Schwarzer R (ed.) Self-efficacy: Thought Control of Action. Washington DC: Hemisphere Publishing.

Bandura A (1997) Self-efficacy: The Exercise of Control. New York. Freeman.

British Thoracic Society (BTS) (1997) British Thoracic Society Guidelines for the Management of COPD. Thorax S2 (supplement 5): 1–28.

Cossette S, Levesque L (1993) Care giving tasks as predictors of mental health of wife caregivers of men with Chronic Obstructive Pulmonary Disease. Research in Nursing and Health 16: 251–263.

Doll R, Peto R, Wheatley K et al. (1994) Mortality in relation to smoking: 40 years' observations on male British doctors. British Medical Journal 309(6959): 901–911.

Engel GL (1977) The need for a new medical model: a challenge for biomedicine. Science 196(4286): 129–135.

Flesch RF (1948) A new readability yardstick. Journal of Applied Psychology. Vol 32 (June): 221–233.

Halpin DMG (2001) Chronic Obstructive Pulmonary Disease. Oxford: Harcourt Publishers.

Hanson EI (1982) Effects of chronic lung disease on life in general and on sexuality: perceptions of adult patients. Heart and Lung: the Journal of Critical Care 11(5): 435–441.

Jacobson E (1929) Progressive Relaxation. Chicago: University of Chicago Press.

Jones PW, Quirk FH, Baveystock CM et al. (1992) A self-complete measure of health status for chronic airflow limitation. The St George's Respiratory Questionnaire. American Review of Respiratory Disease 145(6): 1321–1327.

Krall Scherer Y, Schmieder LE (1997) The effect of a pulmonary rehabilitation programme on self-efficacy perception of dyspnoea and physical endurance. Heart and Lung: the Journal of Critical Care 26(1): 15–23.

McSweeney AJ, Labuhn KT (1990) Chronic Obstructive Pulmonary Disease. In: Spilker B (ed.) Quality of life assessments in clinical trials. New York. Raven Press.

Ogden J (1996) Health Beliefs. In: Ogden J (ed.) Health Psychology: a textbook. Buckingham: Open University Press.

Prochaska JO, Diclemente C (1983) Stages and processes of self-change of smoking: towards an integrative model of change. Journal of Consulting and Clinical Psychology 51(3): 390–395.

Prochaska JO, Diclemente C, Norcross JC (1992) In search of how people change: applications to addictive behaviors. American Psychologist 47(9): 1102–1114.

Randall Curtis J, Deyo RA, Hudson LD (1996) Health related quality of life among patients with COPD. In: Simonds AK, Muir JF, Pierson DJ (eds.) Pulmonary Rehabilitation. London: British Medical Journal Publishing Group.

Salkovskis PM, Warwick HMC (1986) Morbid preoccupations, health anxiety and reassurance: a cognitive-behavioural approach to Hypochondriasis. Behaviour Research and Therapy 24(5): 597–602.

Schrier AC, Dekker FW, Kaptein AA et al. (1990) Quality of life in elderly patients with chronic non-specific lung disease seen in family practice. Chest 98(4): 894–899.

Snaith RP, Zigmond AS (1994) The Hospital and Anxiety and Depression Scale Manual. Windsor: NFER-Nelson.

Sutton K, Cooper M, Pimm J et al. (1999) Anxiety in COPD. The role of illness specific catastrophic thoughts. Cognitive Therapy and Research 23(6): 573–585.

Toshima MT, Kaplan RM, Ries AL (1992) Self-efficacy expectations in chronic obstructive pulmonary disease rehabilitation: self-efficacy in COPD. In: Schwarzer R (ed.) Self-efficacy: Thought Control of Action. Washington, DC: Hemisphere.

Tregonning M, Langley C (1999) Chronic obstructive pulmonary disease. Elderly Care 11(7): 21–25.

van Manen JG, Bindels PJE, Dekker FW et al. (2002) Risk of depression in patients with chronic obstructive pulmonary disease and its determinants. Thorax 57(5): 412–416.

Ware J, Snow K, Kosinski M et al. (1993) SF36 Health Survey Manual: Manual and Interpretation Guide. The Health Institute, New England Medical Centre: Boston, Massachusetts.

Wigal JK, Creer TL, Kotses H (1991) The COPD self-efficacy scale. Chest 99(5): 1193–1196.

Yohannes AM, Baldwin RC, Connolly MJ (2000) Mood disorders in elderly patients with chronic obstructive pulmonary disease. Reviews in Clinical Gerontology 10(2): 193–202.

Zigmond AS, Snaith RP (1983) The Hospital Anxiety and Depression Scale. Acta Psychiatrica Scandinavia 67(6): 361–370.

Chapter 7
Nursing and respiratory care at home

J. SCULLION

Introduction

With an increasingly elderly population, the prevalence of chronic respiratory diseases will increase. In less than 20 years' time, chronic obstructive pulmonary disease (COPD) will be one of the five leading medical burdens on society worldwide (Lopez and Murray 1998). Around 30,000 deaths annually are linked to this disease, yet it is perhaps the morbidity of the condition that has the greatest effect on health care resources, patients and their carers (Halpin 2001). COPD results in frequent consultations in primary care with the average general practitioner having around 200 patients with COPD, of whom 50 will consult, 20 will have acute exacerbations, five will be admitted to hospital and one or two will die (Halpin 2001). This, coupled to a greater pressure to reduce hospital costs leading to earlier discharge of patients and greater severity of illness at time of discharge, means that the focus of respiratory care will increasingly be within the primary-care sector and in particular in the patient's home. This chapter looks at the contribution of health care professionals to respiratory care at home, and in particular the care of the patient with chronic asthma and COPD as this patient group are amongst those most handicapped by their disease, but it is also applicable to patients with many other chronic respiratory conditions.

Chronic respiratory disease leads to increasing impairment, disability and handicap (WHO 1995). Because of the irreversible nature and progressive deterioration of these diseases, the aim of treatment is not curative but to reduce symptoms and in so doing improve health status. The effective care of the chronic respiratory patient involves putting into practice the lessons learnt through pulmonary rehabilitation.

A substantial proportion of the care of the respiratory patient in their own home involves practical advice and support. All patients with a chronic respiratory disease have a limited amount of energy; so it is important to decide with the patient what is important to the patient and how and when to do it.

An effective multidisciplinary team approach can improve patient care by effectively and efficiently dealing with chronic conditions. The partnership between primary and secondary health care teams needs to be strengthened to tackle the impact that chronic respiratory diseases have on patients and on health care resources.

History and assessment

Although the patient with a chronic respiratory condition may have been assessed in general practice and also in the acute hospital setting, it is worth reassessing the patient in the home setting. This is because patients who may appear to be managing their condition well at consultations may be experiencing problems in their own home settings that are remediable. Also, owing to the progressive nature of the diseases, reassessment is useful as the patient's needs may alter over time.

Assessing how the patient perceives their condition is important; it allows the assessment of general well-being and also of the effectiveness of medical treatments. Many patients have effectively ignored their condition for many years, putting symptoms down to the ageing process or seeing them as inevitable because of previous smoking habits. They may therefore have a very negative view of their disease and an element of denial. Although the use of disease-specific questionnaires can be useful in monitoring progress, the patient's own assessment can often be a reliable indicator of their response to treatment and more practical advice.

Education

Education will be important for the patient, no matter what the stage of their disease. This may involve explanation of their disease process, the use and purpose of their medication, and how to maintain health and independence. Advice can be given at regular intervals about lifestyle changes and the importance of both exercise and maintaining independence.

All education and advice will need repeating at regular intervals to ensure that the message is taken on board. It will also need adapting as the patient's condition deteriorates or during times of crisis or exacerbation.

Smoking cessation

Smoking cessation requires an empathetic approach. It is the single most effective treatment for altering outcomes in patients at all stages of COPD (Halpin 2001). Interestingly, patients often put their worsening symptoms down to the fact that they gave up smoking, and many continue to smoke despite advice. Smoking-cessation advice should be given to all patients at every opportunity. There is evidence that successful quitters list advice from a health care professional as one of the main motivational factors for stopping smoking and even brief advice can significantly improve quit rates (Halpin 2001). Advice on nicotine-replacement therapy, or bupropion, when used with psychological support has been shown to improve cessation rates (West 2000).

Some patients may have been refused oxygen or lung volume reduction surgery (LVRS) in light of the fact that they have continued to smoke, and some will have been prescribed oxygen and need to be made aware of the potential risks if they continue to smoke. For patients who have given up smoking yet whose carers continue to smoke, advice for these will be an important factor in the total care package.

Medication

There is at present no drug therapy that had been shown to modify the disease progression in COPD; so the aim of treatment is therefore symptom control. Patients with COPD report a number of symptoms, principal amongst these is breathlessness that in more severe patients occurs on minimal exertion and on undertaking very simple everyday tasks. It is often breathlessness that encourages the patient to seek medical help; unfortunately by this time the damage is irreversible. Other symptoms that patients report include cough, sputum production and wheeze. Patients may also report disturbed breathing patterns, particularly at night when lung function is sub-optimal, increased vagal tone being a likely reason for the increased nocturnal bronchoconstriction.

Many patients, although they do not have a reversible component to their COPD, will derive some symptomatic benefit from bronchodilators. Anticholinergics and beta-2 agonists may improve symptom control. Some patients may respond to Theophylline derivatives, but these work within a narrow therapeutic range, and the side effects should be considered when used in the elderly. Only around 10 to 20 per cent COPD patients show a positive response to steroids (Gross 1995). However, many COPD patients like the effect of steroids, they wake them up, give them an appetite and increase general well-being, and the health care professional should be aware of frequent requests for steroids. For any chronic patient the side effects of corticosteroids, especially oral usage, should be considered and monitored.

There is increasing evidence that the long-acting beta-2 agonists are useful in COPD. Although they work in a similar way to the short-acting beta-2 agonists, they have a longer duration of action (around 12 hours). The long-acting beta-2 agonists improve FEV_1 by up to 200 ml, which may be extremely significant to a breathless patient as well as improving health status and breathlessness (Jones and Bosh 1997). There is also evidence that they reduce exacerbation rates, although the mechanism for this is unclear and may be due to a reduction in breathlessness which leads to a reduced recognition of exacerbations (Halpin 2001). Long-acting anticholinergics and mucolytics may also have a role for specific patients (NCCCC 2004). The NCCCC recommends the choice of drug(s) should take into account the patient's response to a trial of the drug, the drug's side effects, patients' preferences and cost (NCCCC 2004).

Home nebulizer use is controversial and should be initiated only following expert assessment (O'Driscoll 1997). The majority of patients can manage effectively with metered dose inhalers (MDIs) and spacers (O'Driscoll 1997). However, for patients, the use of a nebulizer carries with it a large psychological component in addition to the moistening or cooling effect of the nebulized medication.

The problem with nebulizer treatment is that there are increased drug costs, maintenance may be a problem, and systemic side effects are magnified. Patients' preferences for a nebulizer are very difficult to separate from subjective assessment, making it difficult to assess objectively (Halpin 2001).

Compliance/concordance

Compliance – or, as it is more commonly known now, concordance – is the key to the management of any chronic disease and allows effective management of the condition. Patients appreciate clear instructions on how their medication works, how and when to take their medication, and what to do if symptoms worsen. In looking at a patient's medication, there is a requirement to check dose regimens, whether the patient can take the medication, and that it is in suitable dispensers, and it is useful to check other medication that may be taken (especially over-the-counter medication). The elderly are especially prone to taking over-the-counter preparations that may have an adverse effect on their prescribed medication or, indeed, may exacerbate their symptoms, e.g. non-steroidal anti-inflammatory drugs.

Vaccination

Patients should be encouraged to have influenza and pneumococcal immunization. Annual vaccination of patients with COPD against influenza has been shown to reduce hospital admissions, hospital attendance and death rates (Gorse et al. 1997, Nichol et al. 1999). Pneumococcal vaccination reduces the incidence of invasive pneumococcal disease in patients and has been assessed as cost-effective (Nichol et al. 1999, Franzen 2000).

Osteoporosis

Osteoporosis is a significant problem in patients with advanced COPD. A compounding factor is that patients often experience frequent exacerbations, and the only treatments available are oral steroids and/or antibiotics. Patients may therefore receive far more than the recommended dose of

7.5 mg of steroids over three months (Royal College of Physicians 1999). There is also the problem that COPD patients attribute the feeling of well-being produced by steroids with significant benefit to themselves so will often pressure their general practitioner for repeated courses. Effective treatments and prophylaxis for osteoporosis include calcium and vitamin D, hormone replacement where appropriate, calcitonon and bisphosphonates (Biskobing 2001).

Oxygen therapy

As respiratory function diminishes, the levels of oxygen in the blood may fall. This will lead to increasing breathlessness and also initiates changes in the pulmonary circulation, which can lead to pulmonary hypertension and Cor Pulmonale. If oxygen can be maintained at near-normal levels, the changes to the pulmonary system do not occur and mortality can be significantly reduced. Pulse oximetry is simple to perform in the patient's home, and oxygen saturations of above 92 per cent indicate that the patient is able to maintain their oxygen levels at rest. Unfortunately, oxygen is often prescribed wrongly or inappropriately. Figure 7.1 shows a flow diagram approach to the assessment of oxygen.

Early trials in oxygen therapy showed that using low-concentration oxygen for over 15 hours a day could significantly reduce three-year mortality from 66 to 45 per cent (Medical Research Council 1981). The use of long-term oxygen therapy (LTOT) entails a rate of 2–4 litres delivered by a concentrator, which at this rate gives an inspired concentration of about 24 per cent. The patient can use either a mask or nasal cannula. Cannulae make it easier for patients to eat, drink and talk and may be more comfortable. Only hypoxic patients benefit from oxygen, but many COPD patients will equate the use of oxygen, if they have ever been in hospital, with recovery and feeling better so may feel that they would benefit from oxygen. Some patients benefit from supplementary oxygen if they desaturate on exercise. In the palliative stages of chronic respiratory disease, oxygen may be prescribed for symptomatic relief.

The health care professional, in caring for the patient in their own environment, will need to give advice on oxygen usage and storage. Usage is important as cylinders are expensive and impractical for long-term use. If a patient uses 21 cylinders a month, a concentrator is less expensive to prescribe and normally can be fitted within four working days. Patients can be reassured that the cost of running the concentrator can be reclaimed quarterly. The provision of portable oxygen cylinders allows the patient who requires oxygen to maintain some degree of independence outside of the home.

Exacerbations

Given the nature of chronic respiratory disease, many patients experience acute episodes or exacerbations. The aim of caring for an exacerbation is

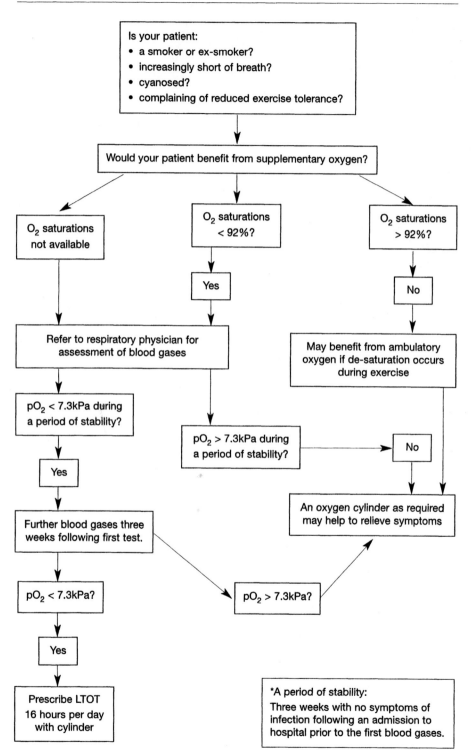

Figure 7.1 Oxygen flow diagram for patients with chronic respiratory problems.

to recognize symptoms, treat any infection, hasten recovery and hospitalize the patient if necessary (Halpin 2001). There is limited evidence for the efficacy of antibiotics in acute exacerbations, although patients often associate them with infections (Snow et al. 2001). Increased breathlessness, a change in sputum colour and/or volume, and wheeze are common symptoms of an exacerbation, and antibiotic use is perhaps most useful when a patient has evidence of two or three of the first three symptoms (Anthonisen et al. 1987).

Given the nature of the disease, COPD, where possible, should be managed at home unless the patient is in a poor condition, experiences deterioration, or there is a general inability to cope (either patient- or carer-based) (British Thoracic Society 1997).

Hospital referral criteria

The criteria for referral of exacerbations to hospital are:

- cyanosed
- severe peripheral oedema
- severe breathlessness
- impaired consciousness
- rapid deterioration
- unable to cope at home
- on LTOT
- poor physical function
- no carer, or carer cannot cope.

There are now many services around the UK offering prompt advice, evaluation and support for patients in the home setting (Killen and Ellis 2000, Gravil et al. 1998, Skwarska et al. 2000). Recent studies have shown that 'hospital at home' schemes for acute exacerbations are safe and a cost-effective alternative to hospitalization (Cotton et al. 2000, Skwarska 2000). However, the preference of both patient and carer to receive care at home is important. A recent randomized controlled trial determined that patients and carers preferred hospital at home to hospital care (Ojoo 2002). However, the very nature of living with a chronic respiratory condition means that patients may get distressed or frightened and feel that they cannot manage at home. Also, carers may sometimes need the break that hospital gives them, and there is limited availability for respite or hospice care. The personal costs of being a carer should never be underestimated.

Patients with an exacerbation should be admitted according to BTS guidelines (NCCCC 2004). A recent King's Fund Survey looking at the pressure on the acute sector over the winter period found that better primary-care management of respiratory conditions, accounting for the majority of excess winter admissions, could have prevented many admissions (Damiani and Dixon 2002). Many breakdowns in the patient's ability to cope at home are because of a lack of adequate support at home, and this will increase the number of acute hospitalizations (Halpin 2001).

Breathlessness

Of all the symptoms that patients with chronic respiratory disease experience, breathlessness is the most commonly reported and the most frightening and limiting for the patients. In one study of patients with chronic respiratory disease, 82 per cent perceived breathlessness as a big problem in their daily lives (Williams 1989). Breathlessness has perhaps the biggest effect on the patient's ability to carry out their normal activities of daily living (ADLs).

However, the degree and impact of breathlessness is not necessarily indicative of the severity of the underlying disease. Many patients with severe disease do not seem to experience breathlessness, yet others at a milder stage of the disease process will be acutely aware of their breathing and experience breathlessness and the accompanying sensations on relatively minimal exertion. Often it is the fear of becoming breathless that leads to inactivity, which in turn leads to deconditioning, anxiety, a loss of independence, helplessness and reduced self-esteem.

Useful home treatments for patients to manage breathlessness, if not covered by a pulmonary rehabilitation programme, are relaxation, physiotherapy and the involvement of occupational therapists (OTs) who can work with the patient on individual goal-setting, including home ergonomics. The patient may need assessment for home aids, such as perching stools, helping hands, bath and stair rails, chair lifts, etc. An OT assessment in the patient's own home may allow the patient to manage their condition within the home setting without having to consider moving to a bungalow, flat or sheltered accommodation. Home helps, through social services, may assist with cleaning and shopping, and panic alarms or mobile phones are also useful so that patients do not feel isolated if alone. Other patients may be in unsuitable accommodation and will need help and support in deciding on an alternative. Any discussion of moving needs to be handled sensitively as many people are very reluctant to move from their family home, however unsuitable it may be.

Anxiety and depression

The nature of COPD would appear to indicate that depression is a common emotional factor (Borak 1991, Light 1985). Depression affects quality of life and will also affect emotional, social and physical functioning (Manen et al. 2000). Although studies investigating depression in COPD are not conclusive due to methodological flaws, most reports suggest higher levels of depression compared with healthy subjects (Borak 1991, Light 1985, Nicholas and Leuner 1992), and Manen et al. (2000) found that for patients with severe COPD the risk of depression was more than doubled.

Studies on anxiety levels in patients have reached similarly inconclusive results. Karajgi et al. (1990) found 16 per cent of patients with COPD had anxiety disorder, yet McSweeny et al. (1982) found 34 per cent and Light et al. (1985) only 2 per cent. Given the chronic nature of COPD, depression would appear to be a reasonable psychological response to the increasing limitations of the disease. What is important is to recognize depression in patients and to determine whether it is reactive and a natural reaction, or endogenous and an underlying disorder to be treated accordingly.

Recognizing depression

Clinical features of depression:

- crying and prolonged sadness
- loss of interest in and loss of enjoyment of life
- poor attention and concentration
- low self-esteem and ideas of worthlessness
- a bleak view of the future and the world in general
- poor sleep and appetite.

Anxiety and depression are linked with breathlessness. Breathlessness leads to anxiety, which in turn leads to over breathing and consequently breathlessness, the so-called 'panic cycle' (Figure 7.2).

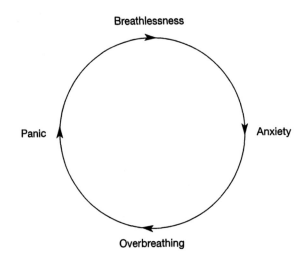

Figure 7.2 The panic cycle.

What is clear is that the experience of breathlessness is extremely distressing and patients can be taught to recognize these feelings and how to control them. In addition to depression and anxiety, COPD is often associated with a poor body image, loneliness, reduced social support, and negative self-concepts (Nicholas and Leuner 1992, Keele-Card 1993). Patients often appreciate having time to talk through some of these issues; however, if the health care professional is unable or unwilling to discuss these issues, referral to a psychologist or counsellor may be appropriate if the patient wishes.

Nutrition

Nutrition should be an important part of the overall care of patients with COPD. Approximately one-quarter of all COPD patients weigh less than 90 per cent of their ideal (Muers and Green 1993). Many patients lose weight, and it is these patients who have an increased mortality (Halpin 2001).

It is unclear what causes the weight loss in COPD, although the pattern of loss is similar to that seen in malignant disease. Patients often have reductions in subcutaneous fat and muscle mass, but there are not often vitamin deficiencies, and levels of circulating protein are often normal. It is possible that the weight loss is due to a combination of factors, such as an increased metabolic demand from the effort of breathing, reduced dietary intake owing to breathlessness and swallowing difficulties. Patients may have a loss of interest in food preparation and lack enjoyment of food. Weight loss appears to have systemic causes similar to the cachexia seen in malignant disease. These factors combine to make malnourishment very difficult to treat in COPD patients; so early detection and treatment are important.

Weight measurement is an important factor in COPD care and can be recorded simply as the patient's body mass index (BMI):

$$\text{BMI} = \frac{\text{weight (in kg)}}{\text{height (in metres}^2)}$$

The results can then be checked against a standard table and the figure documented in the patient's notes (Table 7.1).

Table 7.1 BMI Nutritional Status Table

BMI	Nutritional status
<16	severe malnourishment
16–18.5	moderate malnourishment
18.5–21	at risk
21–25	ideal
25–30	moderate obesity
>30	severe obesity

It is important to remember that the disease also has systemic side effects, oxidative stress, abnormal levels of circulating cytokines, an increase in inflammatory cells and reduced skeletal mass. As the disease prevalence increases with age, it is likely that patients have other medical problems, which will also need to be addressed. Patients who are overweight may find that this increases their breathlessness, so dietary advice for overweight patients is as important as it is for those who are underweight.

Sexuality

One issue often not discussed with patients is that of their relationships or sexuality. Patients with lung disease can become so wrapped up in their illness that they neglect their personal relationships (Scullion 2003). Sexual problems are not in themselves life threatening, but they can cause a great deal of distress to patients, which will affect their quality of life (Gregory 2000).

Chronic lung disease not only affects the sexual act itself but also the individual's sexuality in the wider sense, and too often in the chronic respiratory patient this can be exacerbated by problems with ageing, attitudes and breathlessness (Scullion 2000). The intimacy of a relationship may be important to everyone, but, for the patient with a chronic lung disease, sexual intimacy can sometimes be a very powerful antidote to the depression and isolation that too often results from chronic illness (Hodgkin et al. 1993).

It would appear that there is very little connection between physiological and psychological functioning. An important part of the care of patients should include addressing the psychological and social factors that may affect patients. This may include addressing relaxation skills and giving information on relevant issues such as relationships and sexuality.

Although breathlessness is a major symptom of lung disease, studies have shown that this is not a major problem unless there is breathlessness at rest (Thompson 1986, Fletcher and Martin 1982). Although the act of lovemaking may increase the breathing rate, the physical stress of lovemaking is comparable to climbing 1–2 flights of stairs; although it has to be recognized that styles of lovemaking can vary considerably (Bohen et al. 1984). The effort required for lovemaking does not raise the blood pressure, heart rate or respiration rate to a level that could be considered dangerous.

The person with a chronic respiratory condition will sooner or later experience breathlessness during sexual intimacy. For many patients, the fear of becoming short of breath may lead to the avoidance of sexual activity or an inability to maintain sexual arousal. The partner of a patient with chronic respiratory disease may also believe that abstaining from sexual activity is in the patient's best interests. Nevertheless, maintaining intimacy and closeness with the partner can help to decrease the loneliness and isolation of the person with chronic respiratory disease (The Lung Association 2002).

Sexual relationships concerns may be common, but are often poorly recognized. Often, giving information to patients is enough. If the matter is raised, the subject should always be handled with sensitivity, privacy, and referral if necessary. Problems with lovemaking may be indicative of problems within the relationship, so referral to specialist therapists may help.

A commonsense guide to lovemaking (Scullion 2000):

- when rested
- slowly and surely
- after oxygen and medication
- altering positions
- working on the relationship side
- using all the senses
- experimenting
- late morning or early afternoon
- romance
- avoiding alcohol, heavy meals and cigarettes
- recognizing that orgasm is not the only goal.

Patients can also be advised to avoid sexual positions that put pressure on the chest area and to discover less energy-consuming positions. It is also useful for the able-bodied partner to assume a more active role during lovemaking.

The effects of medication on the libido may be a useful starting point for a discussion about relationships. Medication may be the source of the problem or may be an aggravating factor. Common culprits of impotence and reduced libido include antihypertensives, steroids, Theophylline derivatives and anticholinergics. As many of the patients with chronic respiratory disease have systemic disease and take a lot of medications, it is worth reviewing all prescription and over-the-counter medications. While medication may be the solution to the physical problem, it will not provide the whole answer unless psychological and relationship difficulties have been addressed (Gregory 2000).

Simply touching, being touched and being close to someone is essential to help a person feel loved, special and essentially a partner in the relationship. The patient and the partner are both sexual beings, and the biggest enemy of sexual health is lack of communication (Scullion 2003). Both partners need to agree, and although counselling, support and advice may be given to the patient, any relationship involves agreement between both partners on what is important to them.

Sexuality is an integral and important part of the human experience, and the health care professional needs to be aware of this when trying to address patients' concerns. In dealing with a patient's concerns, health care professionals have to be aware of their role, know how far to go, and when to ask for help (Francoeur 1988).

Health care professionals are advised to get a copy of *Loving Relations*, a simple booklet outlining many of the points discussed above. It is available from jane.scullion@uhl-tr.nhs.uk

Psychosocial support

Although symptom control is a substantial element in the care of chronic respiratory diseases, failure to address other aspects of the patient's life, such as behavioural responses, thoughts about their disease and lifestyle and social and environmental factors, will lead to problems in coping and adapting to the disease. Social support is an important part of human interaction, and patients with a strong support network are likely to have an enhanced health status and quality of life in comparison with someone without any social support. High-risk patients with low social support were found in a study to have significantly more hospitalizations than low-risk patients or patients at high risk with increased social support (Jensen et al. 1994). For some patients, the health care professional may be the focus of support, yet there is little funding available for this to be given to many patients.

The aim of psychosocial support is to:

- minimize the impact of the patient's disease on their lifestyle
- give support and reinforce the patient's own coping mechanisms
- allow for a degree of optimism and hope
- encourage the patient to use anxiety and panic-management techniques
- encourage independence
- maximize the patient's potential.

Patients with COPD can feel that they have failed. At a time in their lives when many should be looking forward to retirement, they find themselves with a chronic disease that does not improve, and in fact progressively deteriorates. This affects not only the patients but also their partners and families. Patients can also suffer from feelings of guilt that they have brought the disease upon themselves due to actions such as smoking, and this unresolved guilt adds further pressure to their psychological overload.

It is often the losses that patients face that are important to them. In addition to the loss of their health, they may have lost their career, their independence, their role, their responsibilities, their relationship and their hobbies.

Palliative care

From the moment of diagnosis, COPD is essentially a terminal disease, and palliation should be important throughout the patient's care.

Palliative care is important in COPD. What is often disregarded with reference to the COPD patient is that this is an essentially terminal disease with the patient experiencing a slowly declining physical functioning that carries with it a concomitant effect on psychosocial function.

> Palliative care is the active, total care of patients whose disease is not responsive to curative treatment. The goal of palliative care is the best quality of life for patients and their families. (WHO 1995)

> There is inadequate provision of palliative care with 75% of people in the UK dying of non-malignant disease but with 95% of the palliative care resources going to cancer patients. (NCHSP 1995)

Patients fear breathlessness and often feel that they are going to die struggling for breath. The sensation of breathlessness is individual and derives from physiological, psychological, social and environmental factors that cause secondary physiological and behavioural responses (Anonymous 1999). If the patient is anxious, it is relevant to use Benzodiazepines to control this. Dihydrocodeine, oral and parenteral opioids have a role in breathlessness and should be given on a trial basis (Jennings et al. 2003). There is currently no supporting evidence for nebulized opioids. Some practitioners may worry about addiction, but in patients with a chronic disease that is essentially terminal in nature it is probably of little consequence.

What is evident is that patients with COPD frequently use somatic complaints to cover their emotional concerns (Kaplan et al. 1993). Taking time to listen to a patient's concerns can sometimes help in alleviating symptoms.

Social factors

It has been found that 44 per cent of deaths from respiratory disease are associated with social-class inequalities (BTS 2002). Social factors such as housing are important for patients' abilities to cope at home and for their general and mental well-being.

Breathe Easy groups offer the patient social support and the opportunity to benefit from group interactions. For patients unable to attend meetings, newsletters and telephone helplines may be available. Local Age Concern groups and volunteers may also be available to offer support to patients, although these vary in availability from area to area.

Benefits

Simple help with benefits advice and applications for 'Blue Badges' help with patients' independence and will have a positive effect on their quality of life. The Benefits Agency has a helpline to discuss what benefits may be available.

End-of-life decisions

End-of-life decisions is an area that is useful to discuss with patients with a chronic disease. Discussions over mortality are not easy; yet for the patient aware of their declining function there may come a time when it is appropriate to allow the subject to be raised. Patients may need to plan for the future and some may wish to consider a 'living will'. Discussion may centre on whether a supportive intervention, such as non-invasive positive pressure ventilation (NIPPV) or intensive therapy unit (ITU) would be appropriate, or comfort and palliation are more appropriate. A study on patient preferences regarding treatment for terminal illness found preference was significantly affected by the burden of therapy in relation to the outcome and the probability of the outcome being positive (Fried et al. 2002).

Effect on carers

As COPD is a chronic progressive disease, patients should be assisted to function as well as possible within the constraints of their condition. Adaptation to the disease is important, while maintenance of a good quality of life is paramount. Besides the cost of the disease to the patient, there is also a huge cost to families and partners. The burden of care usually falls on the family, which needs practical support and efficient social services provision. For some families, the strain of caring may be too much and they will themselves require medical help or may be unwilling or unable to care. Although few areas run carers' groups, these can be beneficial to carers, who may become as isolated as the patient and who may appreciate a break for a few hours a week with others in similar positions.

Conclusion

When caring for the chronic respiratory patient at home, it is often the little changes that can have a dramatic effect on the patient's quality of life. By and large, the majority of chronic respiratory patients uncomplainingly accept their lot in life. They can be a very rewarding group of patients to work with. Unfortunately, patients often hear from health care professionals that there is nothing else that can be done. In this they are wrong. In the words of Trevor Clay, late General Secretary of the Royal College of Nursing, 'There is always something that can be done.'

References

Anonymous (1999) Dyspnea, mechanisms, assessment, and management: a consensus statement. American Thoracic Society. American Journal of Respiratory and Critical Care Medicine 159(1): 321–340.

Anthonisen NR, Manfreda J, Warren CP et al. (1987) Antibiotic therapy in exacerbations of chronic obstructive pulmonary disease. Annals of Internal Medicine 106(2): 196–204.

Biskobing DM (2001) COPD and osteoporosis. Chest 121(2): 609–620.

Bohen JG, Held JP, Sanderson MO et al. (1984) Heart rate, rate-pressure product and oxygen uptake during four sexual activities. Archives of Internal Medicine 144(9): 1745–1748.

Borak J, Sliwinski PP, Piasecki Z et al. (1991) Psychological status of COPD patients on long-term oxygen therapy. European Respiratory Journal 4(1): 59–62.

British Thoracic Society (BTS) (1997) Guidelines for the management of chronic obstructive pulmonary disease. The COPD Guidelines Group of the Standards of Care Committee of the BTS. Thorax 52(supplement 5): S1–S32.

British Thoracic Society (BTS) (2002) The Burden of Lung Disease. http://www.brit-thoracic.org.uk/pdf/BTS

Cotton MM, Bucknall CE, Dagg KD et al. (2000) Early discharge for patients with exacerbations of chronic obstructive pulmonary disease: a randomised controlled trial. Thorax 55(11): 902–906.

Curtis JR, Deyo RA, Hudson LD (1994) Pulmonary rehabilitation in chronic respiratory insufficiency. 7. Health-related quality of life among patients with chronic obstructive pulmonary disease. Thorax 49(2): 162–170.

Damiana M, Dixon J (2002) Managing the Pressure (1997–2000). London: The King's Fund.

Fletcher EC, Martin RJ (1982) Sexual dysfunction and erectile impotence on chronic obstructive pulmonary disease. Chest 81(4): 413–421.

Francoeur RT (1988) Sexual components in respiratory care. Respiratory Management 18(2): 35–39.

Franzen D (2000) Clinical efficacy of pneumonococcal vaccination - a prospective study in patients with longstanding emphysema and/or bronchitis. European Journal of Medical Research 5(12): 537–540.

Fried TR, Bradley EH, Towle VR et al. (2002) Understanding the treatment preferences of seriously ill patients. New England Journal of Medicine 346: 1061–1066.

Gorse GJ, Otto EE, Daughaday CC et al. (1997) Influenza virus vaccination of patients with chronic lung disease. Chest 112(5): 1221–1233.

Gravil JH, Al-Rawas OA, Cotton MM et al. (1998) Home treatment of exacerbations of chronic obstructive pulmonary disease by an acute respiratory assessment service. Lancet 351(9119): 1853–1855.

Gregory P (2000) Patient assessment and care planning: sexuality. Nursing Standard 15(9): 31–33.

Gross NJ (1995) Airway inflammation in COPD: reality or myth? Chest 107 (Supplement 5): 210S–213S.

Halpin DMG (2001) COPD. London: Mosby.

Hodgkin J, Conners G, Bell W (1993) Pulmonary rehabilitation. Guidelines to success. Philadelphia, Pa: Lippincott.

Jennings AL, Davies AN, Higgins JPT et al. (2003) Opioids for the palliation of breathlessness in terminal illness (Cochrane Review). In: The Cochrane Library, Issue 1. Chichester: John Wiley & Sons.

Jensen MP, Turner JA, Romano JM (1994) Correlates of improvement in multidisciplinary treatment of chronic pain. Journal of Consulting and Clinical Psychology 62(1): 172–179.

Jones PW, Bosh TK (1997) Quality of life changes in COPD patients treated with salmeterol. American Journal of Respiratory and Critical Care Medicine 155(4): 1283–1289.

Kaplan RM, Eakin EG, Ries AL (1993) Psychosocial issues in the rehabilitation of patients with COPD. In: Casaburi R, Petty TL (eds.) Principles and Practice of Pulmonary Rehabilitation. Philadelphia, Pa: WB Saunders & Company.

Karajgi BR, Rifkin A, Doddi S et al. (1990) The prevalence of anxiety disorders in patients with chronic obstructive pulmonary disease. American Journal of Psychiatry 147(2): 200–201.

Keele-Card G, Foxhall MJ, Barro CR (1993) Loneliness, depression and social support of patients with COPD and their spouses. Public Health Nursing 10(4): 245–251.

Killen J, Ellis H (2000) Assisted discharge for patients with exacerbations of chronic obstructive pulmonary disease: safe and effective. Thorax 55(11): 885.

Light RW, Merrill EJ, Despars JA et al. (1985) Prevalence of depression and anxiety in patients with COPD. Relationship to functional capacity. Chest 87(1): 35–38.

Lopez AD, Murray CC (1998) The global burden of disease: 1990–2020. Nature Medicine 4(11): 1241–1243.

Manen JG, Bindels PJE, Dekkers FW et al. (2000) Risk of depression in patients with chronic obstructive pulmonary disease and its determinants. Thorax 57(4): 412–416.

McSweeny AJ, Grant I, Heaton RK et al. (1982) Life quality of patients with chronic obstructive pulmonary disease. Archives of Internal Medicine 142(3): 473–478.

Medical Research Council Working Party (1981) Long-term domiciliary oxygen therapy in chronic hypoxic cor pulmonale complicating chronic bronchitis and emphysema. Lancet 1(8222): 681–686.

Muers MF (2000) Opioids for dyspnoea. Thorax 57(11): 922–923.

Muers MF, Green JH (1993) Weight loss in chronic obstructive pulmonary disease. European Respiratory Journal 6(5): 729–734.

National Collaborating Centre for Chronic Conditions (NCCCC) (2004) Management of chronic obstructive pulmonary disease in adults in primary and secondary care. Thorax 59 (Suppl 1): 1–232.

National Council for Hospice and Specialist Palliative Care Services (NCHSP) (1995) Specialist Palliative Care: a statement of definitions. Occasional Paper 8. London: National Council for Hospice and Specialist Palliative Care Services.

Nichol KL, Bakem L, Wuorenma J et al. (1999) The health and economic benefits associated with pneumococcal vaccination of elderly persons with chronic lung disease. Archives of Internal Medicine 159(20): 2437–2442.

Nicholas PK, Leuner JD (1992) Relationship between body image and chronic obstructive pulmonary disease. Applied Nursing Research 5(2): 83–84.

O'Driscoll BR (1997) Nebulisers for chronic obstructive pulmonary disease. Thorax 52(supplement 2): S49–S52.

Ojoo JC, Moon T, McGlone S et al. (2002) Patients' and carers' preferences in two models of care for acute exacerbations of COPD: results of a randomised controlled trial. Thorax 57(2): 167–169.

Royal College of Physicians (1999) Osteoporosis clinical guidelines for prevention and treatment. London: Royal College of Physicians.

Scullion JE (2000) Pulmonary rehabilitation: respiratory modular training programme. In Morgan MDLM, Singh SJ, Scullion JE Respiratory Modular Training Programme: Pulmonary Rehabilitation. PACE Image and Print.

Scullion JE (2003) Sex, breathlessness and respiratory disease. Nurse 2 Nurse 3(8): 31–32.

Shamash J (2002) Catching their breath. Nursing Times 98(20): 14.

Skwarska E, Cohen G, Skwarski KM et al. (2000) Randomised controlled trial of supported discharge in patients with exacerbations of chronic obstructive pulmonary disease. Thorax 55(11): 907–912.

Snow V, Lascher S, Mottur-Pilson C (2001) Joint Expert Panel on Chronic Obstructive Pulmonary Disease of the American College of Chest Physicians and the American College of Physicians. American Society of Internal Medicine. Evidence base for management of acute exacerbations of chronic obstructive pulmonary disease. Annals of Internal Medicine 134(7): 595–599.

The Lung Association (2002) Management of COPD. Living with COPD http://www.lung.ca/copd/management/living/sexuality.html

Thompson WL (1986) Sexual problems in chronic respiratory disease. Achieving and maintaining intimacy. Postgraduate Medicine 79(7): 41–4, 47, 50–52.

West R, McNeill A, Raw M (2000) Smoking cessation guidelines for health professionals: an update. Health Education Authority. Thorax 55(12): 987–999.

Williams SJ (1989) Chronic respiratory illness and disability: a critical review of the psychosocial literature. Social Science and Medicine 28(8): 791–803.

World Health Organization (WHO) (1995) Cancer, pain relief and palliative care. Technical Report, Series 804. Geneva: WHO.

Chapter 8
Occupational therapy in pulmonary rehabilitation

P. J. TURNER-LAWLOR

Introduction

Occupational therapy (OT) is now an established and important component of pulmonary rehabilitation. Occupational therapists are part of the multidisciplinary team that is necessary to deliver a full and comprehensive programme to patients with disabling respiratory disease. Historically, OT was not seen as a strong candidate for inclusion in a pulmonary rehabilitation team as emphasis was very much on exercise, an indispensable intervention. However, following a more holistic approach to this group of patients, the need for other expertise has become evident.

Europe has only recently begun to document the inclusion of OT in pulmonary rehabilitation, and the following is one of the earliest recommendations. All the elements of the randomized controlled trial programme of outpatient rehabilitation reported by Bendstrup et al. (1997) are in detail in the European Society Task Force Position Paper (ERS 1997), except for the OT sessions. Bendstrup et al. felt that these OT sessions may have been an important factor in the improvement of activities of daily living scores reported in the study and therefore, in their opinion, OT would be worth considering for inclusion.

In North America, OT has been an important component of the multidisciplinary approach to respiratory care for much longer, and this was well described by a chapter entitled 'Activities of Daily Living' by Shanfield and Hammond (Hodgkin et al. 1984) and a book by Dempster and DeRenne (1985). The latter, written by two occupational therapists, provides a treatment guide to help other occupational therapists and health care professionals to initiate and develop programmes for the treatment of patients with chronic lung disease.

Activity of daily living management has been identified as of primary importance in pulmonary rehabilitation; indeed, Walsh (see chapter 22 in Casaburi and Petty 1993) states that 'Training in ADL is key to all successful rehabilitation'. A more recent book (Morgan and Singh 1997) contains a chapter written by an occupational therapist, providing guidance in such subjects as lifestyle management, relaxation, coping, sex, aids provision, and benefits. It demonstrates that occupational therapists have a variety of skills that can be applied to a variety of interventions. Some are profession specific, such as advising on activities of daily living and energy conservation, while others (such as stress management) could be provided by any of the rehabilitation team with the appropriate skills and training. However, stress related to performing activities of daily living would be part of the OT assessment, with any issues being addressed by the occupational therapist during intervention.

Occupational therapists' vital role in the pulmonary rehabilitation process has involved the contribution of evaluation of treatments and contributing to the evidence-base specific to OT for pulmonary rehabilitation. The need for further research on the role of OT has been highlighted in recent statements on pulmonary rehabilitation (Anonymous 1997).

The use of disease-specific outcome measures and the questioning of OT processes that lead to the execution of well-designed studies are a necessary part of defining the discipline's contribution. This evidence-base is still in the early stages of evolution, but observational, qualitative and quantitative contributions are now emerging.

This chapter is based on the published work of others and on the author's experience of delivering a pulmonary rehabilitation programme with major OT input for eight years. Rehabilitation can be in-patient, out-patient or home-based, but in the UK it is mostly based as an outpatient service. Concentration will be in this area and will include outcome measures and evidence of effectiveness.

Activities of daily living (ADLs)

Patient profile

Any patient with a chronic respiratory disease with perceived restriction in activities important to them in spite of optimal pharmacological intervention may be a candidate for rehabilitation. Most will have chronic obstructive pulmonary disease (COPD), but patients with other obstructive and restrictive conditions have also been shown to benefit (Ando et al. 2003).

There are no specific lung-function criteria for suitability other than that there should be demonstrable impairment and associated disability and handicap. However, the degree of measurable impairment is poorly related to functional activity in COPD patients (Niederman et al. 1991).

Patients with severe sensory or cognitive impairment or unstable cardiac disease are not suitable for most pulmonary rehabilitation programmes and should be referred to an occupational therapist for individual assessment and treatment outside of the pulmonary rehabilitation remit.

Current smoking is not a contraindication to rehabilitation (Singh et al. 1999), although help with cessation should be offered. Close liaison with the smoking-cessation counsellor is necessary to be able to reinforce the information and guidance given and incorporate into any action plan the patients set themselves during goal-setting.

Considerations when assessing a COPD patient

Chronic disease generally leads to a degree of 'normalization'. Often what the patient perceives as normal or due to age may be interpreted by the clinician as the result of the disease process. This may lead to the inaccurate assessment of disability, particularly in the case of older subjects who tend to view participation in activities as gender-role driven and as less appropriate with increasing age (Ostrow and Dzewaltowski 1985). Could this include rehabilitation and be one reason for non-compliance?

However, the results of a study looking at the role of meaning, enjoyment and symptoms in the functional performance of patients with COPD suggest that patients can enjoy their ADLs, performing meaningful activities despite the symptoms of dyspnoea and fatigue (Leidy and Knebel 2000). Therefore, it is important that occupational therapists provide interventions that recognize the role of meaning and enjoyment of activity as they may enhance performance and quality of life in patients with COPD.

So how are ADLs affected over time in this group of patients?

It is recognized that dyspnoeic patients undergo a downward spiral of muscular deconditioning due to exercise avoidance because of unpleasant experiences of breathlessness while carrying out physical activities. As a result, patients may avoid performing some activities for a time, and, if they then try to resume them, further deconditioning has occurred and breathlessness is worse. This sets up a pattern of increasing difficulty with, and the gradual and eventual elimination of, activities from the patient's lifestyle.

In a study comparing activities in categories of home management/domestic ADL, body care/movement and social recreation, COPD patients most frequently eliminated lawn mowing, ironing, auto-repair, home repairs, walking one mile and going out to the pub from their ADLs. These findings highlight the concept that dyspnoea scores remain constant over time because those activities that would increase dyspnoea scores are eliminated.

Keeping in mind that there appears to be no correlation between forced expiratory volume in 1 second (FEV_1) and functional ability, potential benefits from rehabilitation on the ability to perform tasks should not be based on lung-function measurements and pre-rehabilitation assessment alone, but on reassessment immediately following rehabilitation when benefits have been realized (Niederman et al. 1991).

As patterns of activity and inactivity are unique to each individual, categorizing specific activities to declining lung-function measurements is not a good guide to the OT requirements of the COPD patient. This makes the procedure of individual goal-setting and the use of a disease-specific ADL questionnaire imperative so that the planning and implementation of an effective treatment programme during and following pulmonary rehabilitation can take place.

Goal-setting

This is a vital activity in which the patient in conjunction with the therapist sets *realistic* goals to be achieved in the short and long term with the help of rehabilitation. To do this the patient's understanding of their own impairment, disability and handicap is explored before agreed goals are set. The setting of realistic goals leading to improvement in self-esteem is one of the seven factors in a pulmonary rehabilitation programme that seem to be responsible for improved performance and psychological states (Agle et al. 1973).

Practically, to start members of each rehabilitation group thinking about what their realistic goals would be, a pencil and paper exercise can be carried out in session one. It asks the questions: 'What would you like to gain from this course? What are your expectations?' Each member's expectations are then shared and a collective list is drawn up and displayed on a flip chart. This stimulates conversation and, importantly, reminds individuals of areas of difficulty that they had forgotten to mention. Any expectation that is unrealistic, beyond the therapist's control, or out of the remit of the pulmonary rehabilitation programme is at this stage clearly pointed out to the individual(s), thus dispelling any confusion or disappointment later on. This can be reinforced during a one-to-one goal-setting session.

Individual goal setting should take place in a private room as this allows confidentiality and the opportunity to discuss private matters that patients would otherwise find uncomfortable if addressing in a group situation. A mix of physical and psychological short-term goals is encouraged, thus covering every aspect of the patient as an individual coping with a chronic disease. The emphasis is on setting goals that individuals feel will enhance their quality of life and that they can progress towards or achieve by the end of the programme. At least one long-term goal is also encouraged, that the individual would like to see themselves doing in six to 12 months' time. Often this is to be able to go away on holiday again!

Goals relating to ADLs tend to dominate in the patient's selection, with most activities chosen because of the associated breathlessness experienced. The most frequently cited activities among patients from the pulmonary rehabilitation programme at Llandough Hospital are climbing stairs, personal care/hygiene, walking – such as going to the shop to buy a paper or a leisure walk with or without a dog, playing with the grandchildren, and domestic activities that are peculiar to each individual depending on priorities and gender. The individual goal-setting also allows patients to express feelings of reduced confidence, increased anger and frustration, increasing anxiety, depression and fear related to breathlessness and panic. The goal-setting session is an ideal opportunity to be alert to signs of anxiety and depression, which is often undiagnosed in this group of patients. Where anxiety and depression exist, it has been shown they can be improved by pulmonary rehabilitation (Withers et al. 1999, Griffiths et al. 2000).

If the patient attaches an 'importance score' to each goal, priorities can be arrived at. An outcome measure used successfully for goal-setting has been based on the MOTEM (Morriston Occupational Therapy Outcome Measure) (James 2001).

In the final week of the pulmonary rehabilitation programme there should be a goal-achievement feedback session. This can take the form of a group session when all group members have the opportunity to feed back to each other. Being aware of this session from the outset can have the effect of maintaining motivation and drive to progress towards and/or meet set goals by the end of the course. Mutual support from group interaction and all those factors within patients that lead to strong motivation and follow-up to consolidate gains (Agle et al. 1973) are important factors present in this goal-setting process. Group dynamics have a major impact on success. Throughout the programme, patients give each other encouragement, provide a listening ear to each other's progress, and provide an important 'pat on the back' that gives a sense of achievement and self-esteem so often missing in this group of patients. Competitiveness should be discouraged, especially during exercise/activity sessions, with emphasis being placed on individual achievements within the group setting. Opportunity should also be provided for individual feedback for those who have particular goals of a sensitive and private nature not appropriate to sharing in a group session. It is important that the patient and therapist know about this choice at the time they set their goals.

The therapist uses guidance and motivational skills to encourage the patient to take the appropriate steps to change, in other words fulfilling their goals. This is imperative, as readiness to change may improve compliance with physical training/activity (Marcus et al. 1992), which has been shown to have long-term benefits for the patient.

Assessment of ADLs

ADLs may be severely restricted in patients with COPD. Dyspnoea during routine activities leads to significant disability and handicap and so assessment of these two areas is required to evaluate the effect on daily life. A survey of patients with severe COPD showed that 78 per cent had shortness of breath when walking around at home and had difficulty performing routine ADLs (Restrick et al. 1993).

Suitable assessments and outcome measures of ADLs for patients with COPD are now becoming established. Previous OT assessment, particularly in the Llandough programme, was initially based on activities being placed in personal, domestic and work/leisure domains and graded into categories of increasing strenuousness (very light, light, moderate and heavy) according to the oxygen requirement for each task (Hodgkin et al. 1993). Becoming familiar with these categories would be a useful adjunct to improving insight into overall effort required for an ADL. (This will be addressed later.) This homespun ADL questionnaire was completed by the patient and evaluated by the occupational therapist. Problems were identified, appropriate advice and intervention given and, if required, a home visit carried out. However, it became evident over time that the questionnaire did not fulfil the requirements necessary to:

- assess activities in relation to degrees of breathlessness experienced
- evaluate difficulty of activity by having a reliable and repeatable scoring system
- reassess accurately
- have an outcome measure that was disease specific or validated for use with COPD patients
- compare outcomes with other programmes thus evaluating the overall programme and any need for change in the intervention process
- build a validated evidence base of OT intervention for ADLs
- be used in research studies for the benefit of advancing the precise nature of the interventions in pulmonary rehabilitation.

The questionnaires, discussed at the end of this chapter, are now being used successfully in pulmonary rehabilitation programmes in the UK, but to determine which one to use will depend on such factors as:

- **Time**: do you have dedicated hours specifically for pulmonary rehabilitation? Are they enough to allow you to do fuller assessments and the follow-up evaluation/scoring? Do you then have time to reassess as well as carry out the intervention/home visit?
- **Administration support**.
- **Access to a computer** for scoring/recording data.
- **Whether the instrument is to be used as an outcome in a research study** either as part of a battery of secondary outcome tests or if it is to be used as the major outcome of a specific question within the study.
- **Ease of use by the population of patients you are treating**. Literacy, culture, age and cognitive abilities need to be taken into consideration, together with the emotional state of some individuals at the beginning of a programme. Patients might need help filling in the questionnaires and reassurance that pulmonary rehabilitation will assist in improving their abilities if initial despondency is evident. Questionnaires can highlight their growing difficulties with purposeful activity and so can become a negative experience.

ADLs: practical application

OT is primarily aimed at enabling patients to perform the ADLs satisfactorily to them; to this end the OT's aim is to:

- promote economy of movement and effort through:
  - **education** – pacing, coping skills, time management, work efficiency
  - **ergonomics** – posture, reorganization of work areas, comfort
  - **demonstration and supply** of simple aids
- promote and encourage regular exercise as part of the daily routine; improved physical function can then be transferred to performing desired ADLs
- improve activity and ability in the patient's own home environment through:
  - home visits, assessments and liaison with social services and other appropriate agencies.

Economy of movement and effort

The overall effort required for an ADL is expressed in terms of human energy expenditure or cost (Passmore et al. 1955, Ainsworth et al. 1993, Compendium of Physical Activities 2000). Energy conservation is a skill in which patients may be trained during pulmonary rehabilitation to perform activities using the minimum energy expenditure possible. Gilbert (1965), an occupational therapist, incorporated studies of the energy cost of homemaking activities as early as 1965. By reducing the level of energy expenditure and consequently the rate of oxygen consumption, the patient can benefit from decreased feelings of fatigue and breathlessness, and increased comfort.

If a patient is comfortable in an activity, they may be likely to stick with an activity for longer, or even take up one that has been previously eliminated. Some forms of advice that may help to reduce symptoms and increase comfort do not necessarily reduce oxygen consumption but are important in enhancing performance and quality of life. For example, sitting is often suggested during an activity, though the fatigue of standing is related to stresses placed on the circulatory and neuromuscular systems (Larsen 1947). Lower-limb muscles are often weak in COPD patients and can be the cause of cessation of activity before breathlessness becomes a limiting factor. Therefore, beside improved muscle stamina and strength, correct body positioning for working is imperative to maintain comfort.

Other examples of intervention that may increase comfort are the teaching of appropriate breathing techniques (co-ordinating breathing with daily activities has been shown to help (Dempster and DeRenne 1985)) and advice on controlling environmental factors such as dust, fumes, steam and heat. Comfort during activity is necessary to help reduce anxieties and motivate patients into action. 'Activity efficiency' is perhaps an appropriate term to use when describing both energy-conservation techniques and advising on comfort factors that do not necessarily conserve energy.

The overall effort required for an ADL may be reduced by using those muscles that are essential for the task, while those not needed are resting. Another term for this is 'differential relaxation'. Simple examples of this approach might be to teach the use of a perching stool while washing-up or brushing teeth (Bratton 1958); the use of bath aids for getting in and out of the bath; relaxing the hands while talking, and the shoulders and face while typing or driving. Thus the patient is enabled to achieve more of their essential routine activities with less effort and less assistance from others. Time and energy are then left for more enjoyable leisure activities, as opposed to using spare time non-productively to recover, before the next essential chore of the day. Unless tackled efficiently, the problems lead to COPD patients spending large segments of time watching television and adopting a very sedentary and emotionally dependent life.

With help from the occupational therapist, the ergonomics of tasks can be tackled. Patients learn to check their posture in relation to their furniture and work surfaces, making necessary changes to reduce wasted effort (McCracken and Richardson 1959, Ogden and DeRenne 1985).

Seating should be both supportive and allow ease of function. Seating posture should follow the golden rules of bottom well back in the seat, feet on a firm supportive surface, knees at a 90-degree angle, small of back supported and trunk held in an upright position to allow ease of breathing while carrying out an activity. To allow this to happen, the work surface should be at a height in line with the individual's forearms when bent at 90 degrees at the elbows and held out level in front of them. Advice on aids such as an adjustable footstool/step or perching stool to maximize ease of reach, or devices to raise the height of furniture and work surfaces, may help the patient to make small but beneficial adjustments to performance of tasks. Clear, simple information and instructions with diagrams should be available as back-up handouts for patients to refer to at home.

Tasks can be broken down into achievable stages and work areas reorganized to cut down on the effort used, thus maximizing efficiency. A patient's approach to tasks is addressed. They learn to break down the task into small, achievable steps, which can be carried out over an extended period of time depending on the job in hand. For example, washing up a main meal might take an hour because it includes two rest breaks, while a DIY project can be spaced over several days or weeks taking into account the physical and emotional demands of the task and the individual who is carrying it out.

The patient is taught to ask questions about how they would do a given job. These might include:

- 'Are all the necessary materials and equipment available before I start, and, if so, are they in easy reach?'
- 'Are good body mechanics being used?'

- 'How shall I best use my breathing techniques while carrying out the task?'
- 'Can this task be done sitting instead of standing if it does not involve frequent movement from place to place?'
- 'Are the sitting facilities comfortable and of the proper height?'
- 'Can any part of this task be changed, delegated or omitted and still produce the desired results?'
- 'What is my attitude towards this task? Will my like or dislike of the job affect my ability to cope and accomplish it to my satisfaction?'

Reorganization of workspaces can be carried out by following simple guidelines:

- Collect together or locate items near each other when carrying out a task. A good example of this is making a cup of tea, as it involves storage, lifting and carrying activities.
- The ideal level for storing frequently used items is between 28 and 45 inches (71–114 cm) from the floor. Items used every day should be located between shoulder and hip level. It is easier for patients to visualize this instruction rather than giving measurements alone. Individuals may thus adjust their working environment according to their own height and arm reach, using the knowledge of their own home situation.
- Rarely used items should be stored at the highest and lowest level.

The bending, reaching and lifting difficulties, which are often seen in this group of patients, complicate tasks such as dressing, bathing and cleaning. For these activities, simple aids such as a helping hand, sock gutter, bath-board and seat can be used to minimize effort and so reduce breathlessness, fatigue and feelings of anxiety, frustration and anger while increasing speed, efficiency, confidence and independence. These kinds of aids help to conserve energy for carrying out the main part of the task comfortably and often in less time. Other aids, which simply take over a task, such as stair climbing, may increase disability and handicap and confirm a sense of dependency. Reassessment *following* pulmonary rehabilitation is advisable before major recommendations are made, such as installing stair-lifts or domestic building works.

Throughout the rehabilitation programme, patients are taught and encouraged to use pacing skills to manage their time more realistically and effectively (Fontana 1993). Pacing means working slowly and smoothly, developing a pace where the level of dyspnoea remains comfortable and fatigue is minimized by taking rest breaks. Patients must learn the pace that is best for them. When combined with the use of breathing techniques and improved physical fitness, greater mobility around the home environment can be achieved. The use of stairs or steps, and activities such as hanging out the washing, gardening and walking to the local shop to buy a newspaper are encouraged.

Pacing is an important concept in being able to get through the day, with encouragement to take breaks and relax, and not to feel defeated or a failure if a job is not completed all at once, or even on the same day. Communication on this matter with family members, friends or carers is advisable. It must be stressed that they should not step in and take over or finish off a task, even though in their eyes it is taking too long, is not up to their expectations, and/or they *perceive* the patient is not coping. Unless the patient requests assistance, it is best to let them complete the task, otherwise the sense of achievement will be lost, and that will affect continuing improvement and reduce drive and motivation built up during the rehabilitation programme.

Extension of care in pulmonary rehabilitation

A home visit is often an essential part of evaluating a patient's ability to cope and manage their condition. Demonstration by the occupational therapist and practice by the patient with aids in the home provides a realistic picture of physical independence levels. Observation of behaviour patterns in stressful situations, such as prior to climbing the stairs or taking a bath, may reveal why breathlessness or panic is affecting the patient's ability to perform tasks.

However, to provide a seamless service for the COPD patient – which involves following them from the in-patient bed, back into the community during the recovery period of the exacerbation, and to referral for a pulmonary rehabilitation programme – a community team care approach should be adopted. Rehabilitation is therefore part of a continuum of care with interchange of ideas and information with home care teams, which are now being set up to provide more acute care in the patient's home.

I should like to describe a domiciliary service, known as the Community Respiratory Resource Unit. It was formed as a multidisciplinary team of nursing staff, physiotherapist and occupational therapists, with the aim of maximizing quality of life, promoting appropriate use of primary- and secondary-care resources, and of preventing readmission following discharge for this group of patients.

The team members are all trained to do basic physiological measurements, which include:

- blood pressure
- spirometry
- pulse
- weight
- temperature
- pulse oximetry.

They also check the efficiency of inhaler techniques using an electronic device.

A referred patient is assigned a keyworker, who carries out the initial assessment and addresses the patient's immediate problems. The first checks cover medication, inhaler techniques, ensuring that they are stable and safe, and to provide reassurance at every stage of recovery. As the patient improves, very simple, appropriate exercises are provided plus an individualized self-management plan, which includes an action plan if an exacerbation occurs. A copy is sent to both the GP and their consultant on discharge.

The keyworker of the patient provides all the basic education (what is COPD?), advises on stress management and relaxation, work efficiency, exercise and breathing techniques. If, following assessment, specific expertise is required for a particular problem that the keyworker cannot provide, the patient is referred to the appropriate discipline.

The occupational therapist specifically covers ADLs and aids. Advice and handouts are adapted from those used in the pulmonary rehabilitation programme, the aim being to complement the programme content and so prepare the patient for future referral.

Visits are intense, beginning with two to three visits in the first week, each lasting about one hour. There are exceptions when this can rise to five a week if the patient is particularly weak and unwell, anxious and needs lots of reassurance, and if there are difficult social factors. On the other hand, this can fall to one a week if there is good family support, the patient's condition is stable, there is little or no anxiety, and they are already knowledgeable about their condition and its management. Maximum input is for eight weeks before referral to a pulmonary rehabilitation programme and/or formal discharge into the GP's care. Importantly, the team has direct access to clinics, lung function and medical emergency services

This keyworker approach provides a truly unique multidisciplinary structure, which extends further the skills and contribution made by the occupational therapist in respiratory care.

Stress management and relaxation

Patients readily identify situations often unrelated specifically to exertion in which breathlessness, anxiety and panic are encountered (Agle et al. 1977, Smoller et al. 1996). A patient's fear of dyspnoea may lead to avoidance of otherwise achievable physical activity, resulting in physical deconditioning. A related problem is that of poor sleeping patterns, which are not always due to dyspnoea. Difficulty getting to sleep and early-morning waking often stem from the time of formal diagnosis and relate to subsequent anxieties about what the future may hold. Patients may be helped by an understanding of why these problems come about. Techniques of stress management (Anonymous 2001, Ogden and

DeRenne 1985), relaxation and controlled-breathing techniques may be taught, which help to establish an internal locus of control and strategies for coping that do not depend on access to inhaled medication (Renfroe 1988, Broussard 1979, Gift et al. 1992, Gallefoss and Bakke 1999).

Practical application

In stress-management group sessions, the patients can undertake a series of exercises that help them to understand what stress is and what its physical and psychological effects are. Patients then specifically identify their own stressors. These may be a mismatch between perceived demands and perceived ability to cope, and exaggerated emotional responses to the situation. Patients are taught to identify warning signs that indicate to them that they are reaching their fatigue point and so their breathing pattern and control could be affected. Such signs might be increased irritability and anxiety, disrupted sleep and eating patterns, inability to distinguish between minor and major details.

Patients are encouraged throughout to share their concerns, difficulties that they have encountered, and solutions that they have found helpful in coping with their dyspnoea, frustration, disability and handicap. This group interaction provides an effective learning environment for both patients and therapist. Once these issues have been explored, a 'framework for action' is practised (see Figure 8.1) and skills developed to fill up a 'toolbox' with new and improved coping strategies. The patient is, hypothetically, given an empty 'toolbox' at the beginning of the programme, which is gradually filled with useful tools that they can pick from to address the task or need that is specific to them.

These include:

- relaxation techniques
- breathing techniques and postural awareness
- purposeful and functional activity (adopting old or developing new interests)
- assertiveness, positivity and adaptability
- a problem-solving approach to deal with stress during ADLs.

Relaxation

Relaxation plays a major part in helping to fill the 'toolbox', as it is an important part of stress management, which offers different techniques for different situations. Relaxation is a skill, and like any skill it needs to be practised regularly to realize all its benefits. These benefits should be explained clearly during the initial introduction, and be emphasized throughout the programme's practice sessions.

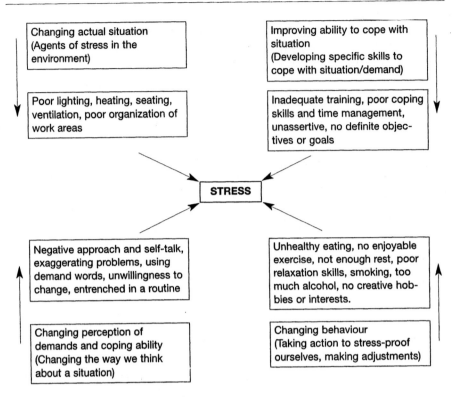

Figure 8.1 Framework for action.

Benefits of relaxation

- a simple and effective way of reducing the stress response
- increases self-awareness of effects of stress on body and mind
- reduces fatigue by increasing awareness of inappropriate muscle tension
- increases confidence in ability to deal with feelings of anxiety and panic
- helps promote calm, controlled breathing
- helps promote feelings of calmness and sense of well-being
- helps promote sleep
- provides an alternative to drugs for the relief of symptoms
- can improve overall performance in daily living skills (differential relaxation)
- can improve personal relationships

Relaxation techniques

- Progressive Relaxation Technique (Jacobson 1938, 1976)
- Deep Relaxation with Breathing Awareness (Madders 1981)
- Guided and Unguided Visualization (Lichstein 1988)

- 'STOP' technique (part of pulmonary rehabilitation programme delivered at Llandough Hospital, UK) (see Figure 8.2)
- Differential Relaxation (Bernstein and Borkovec 1973, Mitchell and Bartlett 1987)

The emphasis is on attaining and maintaining *calm, controlled breathing* with awareness of abdominal movement every time, whatever method is used. Focusing on breathing rhythm can sometimes upset a patient's breath control, and such patients may benefit more from visualization techniques – in which the mind and posture are relaxed, leading unconsciously to a calm breathing pattern. Deep relaxation with breathing awareness technique has the most focus on the experience of calm and controlled breathing. It is often the most useful technique as it takes away the extreme conscious effort of reducing the breathing rate, which is often seen in this group of patients. Patients are encouraged to practise at home to maintain focus. The more they practise, the more effective it becomes. A number of the above techniques should be taught during the course of the programme as this equips the patient to choose the one that best suits their needs at a particular time. Thus, a 20-minute progressive relaxation technique may be selected for muscle tension awareness, or a 30-second 'STOP' technique (Figure 8.2) may be chosen for use in sudden stressful, dyspnoea-provoking situations and help stop the development of anxiety and worry.

Conduct of relaxation sessions

Tapes versus personal instruction:
During pulmonary rehabilitation relaxation sessions, it is best that instruction comes from the therapist as opposed to a cassette tape, as a health care professional is able to gauge the length, speed and rhythm of the delivery according to the patient's reactions. Instructions can be phrased in such a way that participants individually decide on a pace that suits them. This is particularly important in the early stages when patients can be self-conscious and unsure of themselves learning this new skill. Personal instruction, by the therapist, should allow the patient to develop a slower breathing pattern without imposing timings on the phases of the respiratory cycle, which, on most available tapes, are appropriate to people with normal lungs rather than people with COPD.

The therapist can also observe a patient's progress during the session and make adjustments to improve the effect of the method used and record important issues afterwards that can be addressed in the group or with individuals at the next session. Tapes can be useful adjuncts to encourage continuing practice at home. These should preferably be recorded in the unit or recommended by the therapist to complement the programme. Once a patient is skilled at relaxation, relaxing music might be the only stimulus they need to feel a benefit.

Use in emergency situations

WARNING!
Remember: we are most at risk of lapsing into a state of worry/anxiety when we are at rest, doing a routine task that occupies only part of our attention, or thinking ahead about a difficult activity and/or situation.

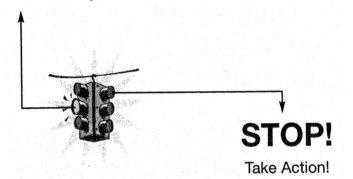

STOP!
Take Action!

- Say very firmly, '**STOP**'. You can say this out loud or to yourself, but it must be said firmly and with conviction.
- Then take a breath in (as much as you feel is comfortable for you).
- Let your breath out as if you were trying to blow out the flame of a small candle. (You can imagine that the flame is the anxiety/worry you are blowing away.)
- Drop your shoulders into a position of ease and relaxation as you breathe out.
- Allow another gentle breath in and then breathe out with a sigh. (It might help to close your eyes while you do this)
- Again, as you breathe out, drop your shoulders further and relax your face by loosening your jaw (check your teeth are not clamped together and your tongue is resting comfortably in the bottom of your mouth).
- If possible, take a small step back to hypothetically distance yourself from your anxiety/worry. When you are ready and feeling more in control, continue with your activity.

To begin with, practise this technique as many times as you can during the course of a day until it becomes familiar and easy to do, so when a real emergency situation arises you can apply it with ease.

Figure 8.2 The 'STOP' technique.

Relaxation summarized

- outward breath
- feeling of calm, controlled breathing
- rise and fall of abdominal muscles
- use of hand gently placed over abdomen to distinguish change of movement
- change in breathing rate – auditory awareness
- feedback following session – awareness of reported difficulties and achievement of sense of relaxation.

Differential relaxation

Differential relaxation can be incorporated into the programme of relaxation training as it can aid the reduction of feelings of breathlessness and fatigue, thus increasing levels of activity and independence. Muscle tension is essential for carrying out purposeful activity; however, when accompanied by tension in muscles that do not benefit the action, such as grimacing and gripping the steering wheel tightly while driving, energy is being used unnecessarily.

Differential relaxation focuses on controlling the levels of muscle tension while the individual is engaged in activity (see 'Economy of movement and effort' above). Since an ability to recognize muscle tension at its varying levels is essential for developing this skill, differential relaxation should be presented after the patient has learnt progressive relaxation which has allowed the patient to identify their own particular tension areas. Recognition and elimination of all unnecessary tension, and of any excessive tension in the muscles performing the activity, is the goal.

Differential relaxation is relatively easy to achieve in activities that do not cause any anxiety, but is more difficult in situations that have become stressful with heightened feelings of breathlessness. Examples of common situations in which anxiety might impede relaxation are in crowded places, such as public transport, shops or at social events, or when a patient experiences feelings of being trapped (physically or emotionally), such as living with COPD or family situations where there are disagreements and over-protectiveness by family members. In such cases, additional strategies may need to be used to reduce excessive tension. Mental rehearsal of an event, and positive self-talk, avoiding exaggeration of the significance of the problem and avoiding the use of demand words such as 'must' and 'should', may be helpful. The use of visualization and breathing control or the 'STOP' emergency technique is also recommended.

Assessment and outcome measures

Disease-specific ADL questionnaires

1: Pulmonary Functional Status and Dyspnoea Questionnaire (PFSDQ)

There are two versions of the PFSDQ, the original long version (Lareau et al. 1994) and the modified version (Lareau et al. 1998). For clinical evaluation there was a need to include activities that:

- crossed the span of energy workloads (Passmore et al. 1955)
- represented self-care activities appropriate for the middle-aged and the elderly
- were performed by male and female patients
- were performed by ambulatory as well as bedridden patients.

The long version is a self-administered questionnaire, which according to the originators should take the patient no longer than 20 minutes to complete. However, many patients may find it can take longer than this and so time allowance should be generous if it is scheduled to be completed during a pulmonary rehabilitation session. Alternatively, the patient can take the questionnaire home to fill in at their leisure and return at the next session.

The questionnaire consists of two components, each involving the same 79 activities. Activities are independently evaluated for ease of performance, as well as with the degree of associated dyspnoea.

A: The **activity level** evaluates the degree to which the patient's ability to perform ADLs has changed as a result of their chest condition. Activities are grouped into six categories:

> self-care (15 items)
> mobility (14)
> eating (8)
> home management (22)
> social (10)
> recreational (10).

Activities are rated on a scale of 1 to 10, with 1 being 'As active as I've ever been' and 10 being ' Have omitted entirely'. Alternatively, the patient may indicate that they have never performed that activity. The latter is valuable information when carrying out goal-setting and intervention, as unnecessary discussion of irrelevant activities can be avoided and scoring can be adjusted so it remains accurate for relevant activities. Not many questionnaires have this scope.

B: The **dyspnoea component** has two aspects. The first asks the patient about their experience of dyspnoea, for example the degree of dyspnoea experienced on most days during the past year or with day-to-day activities. The second aspect measures the level of dyspnoea patients report while performing their ADLs. Activities are rated on a scale of 0, indicating no dyspnoea, to 10, indicating very severe dyspnoea. If it has been established as never having been an activity, it is left without a rating score.

The original research found the PFSDQ a valid and reliable tool for measuring patients' dyspnoea and their ability to perform ADLs. However, its main disadvantage was the length of time it took to complete. Consequently, a modified version was developed.

2: The Modified Pulmonary Functional Status and Dyspnoea Questionnaire (PFSDQ-M)

Like the PFSDQ, the modified version is a self-complete questionnaire and is sensitive to small changes in dyspnoea with activities, as well as activities being independently evaluated for performance. However, there is a third component in addition to activity and dyspnoea, which covers fatigue. Fatigue was added because, after dyspnoea, it is the most common symptom of which patients with COPD complain.

The activity and dyspnoea components are similar to the original PFSDQ, except the number of activities rated is reduced to ten. The fatigue section is divided into two parts: the first asks about their experience of fatigue and the second asks the patient to rate on a scale of 0 (none) to 10 (very severe) the degree of tiredness felt performing each of the ten activities listed.

For both questionnaires, the scoring can be simply done using a calculator. It takes time to begin with, like anything unfamiliar, but, once a pattern and scoring record is established, a valuable outcome measure will emerge. Research has shown that both the original and the modified versions are useful in providing information about patients and how their dyspnoea affects their ability to perform ADLs.

If an assessment tool as well as an outcome measure is required, it is advisable to use the longer version. However, the addition of the fatigue component in the modified version provides valuable information for the occupational therapist when planning and advising on energy-conservation techniques specific to the activities highlighted as being tiring.

An advantage of the PFSDQ is that it identifies not only problems of activity due to breathlessness but also activities affected by other conditions that cause disability and handicap. These, such as osteoporosis (common in COPD patients), rheumatoid or osteoarthritis, can be addressed during the programme alongside their respiratory difficulties.

The questionnaire, with further information gleaned from the goal-setting session, gives greater insight into the needs of each individual. Therefore the occupational therapist can be perceptive to and incorporate these needs into educational and stress management aspects of the overall programme, thus reinforcing information and guidance given on an individual basis. An example, which seems to occur with regularity, is 'social events being omitted entirely'. This can be addressed successfully in a session looking at the perceived ability to cope as opposed to the actual ability, known as the 'transactional model of stress' (Cox 1978). This is generally useful for the entire group, as resulting discussion heightens awareness and understanding that can be acted upon immediately or in the future when occasion arises.

The questionnaire can flag up when many activities have been omitted and the possibility that the family have taken over, whether the patient wished them to or not. Conflict and misunderstanding can arise and the patient's spiral of deconditioning is reinforced unwittingly. If the patient wishes, this can be discussed with their family, who can also be invited to attend educational sessions to help them improve their understanding of the management of COPD.

3: London Chest Activity of Daily Living Scale (LCADL)

This questionnaire has been validated as a new assessment tool of ADLs in patients with severe COPD (mean FEV_1 42 per cent predicted) (Garrod et al. 2000). Data from a small study, by the originators, support the use of the LCADL as an outcome measure in COPD showing reliability (assessed in 14 patients – median age 65) and sensitivity (assessed in 59 patients – median age 66) (Garrod et al. 2002).

It is an administered questionnaire, which is quick and comprehensible. It is a standardized 15-item questionnaire designed to assess routine ADLs. There are four sections covering self-care (4 items), domestic (6), physical (2) and leisure (3). The question asks 'How breathless have you been during the last few days while doing the activities listed?' The response is on a scale of 0 (wouldn't do it anyway) to 5 (someone else does it for me), scoring 1, 2, 3, 4 or 5.

Recent data have been provided to support the sensitivity of the LCADL as a measure of breathlessness in COPD; however, further use and evaluation in pulmonary rehabilitation programmes is encouraged to establish its full potential as an assessment and outcome measure (Garrod et al. 2002). Owing to its particularly short and precise nature aimed at elderly, severe COPD patients, it may have limitations as an assessment tool for other categories of COPD patients. For the occupational therapist to make an accurate evaluation prior to goal-setting, a very full picture of the patient's perception of their ability is necessary. The LCADL assessment appears not to fulfil that particular requirement, but could be valuable as an accompanying outcome measure in evaluating the programme itself.

Non-disease-specific ADL questionnaires

The following measurements were originally designed for assessment of ADL in other conditions but are now being used with COPD patients.

1: Nottingham Extended ADLs Scale (NEADL)

This was originally designed for assessment of ADLs in stroke patients (Nouri and Lincoln 1987, Lincoln and Gladman 1992). Studies have shown that the NEADL questionnaire is able to discriminate between COPD patients with MRC dyspnoeic grades 3/4 and 5 in terms of performance of daily activities and levels of disability (Bestall 1999). Earlier work has shown an association with the NEADL questionnaire and severity of disease (Okubadejo 1997).

It is useful in baseline assessment and post-rehab assessment (Mason et al. 1999). However, a randomized controlled trial concluded that, though useful in baseline assessment, it was insensitive to changes in performance in ADL after a pulmonary rehabilitation programme (Wedzicha 1998). (NB: this was a programme for very severe COPD patients only.)

The NEADL measures the daily activities of the patient during a typical week. It is a short, self-administered questionnaire, which takes 2–4 minutes to complete and consists of 22 items. The items are divided into four subscales covering mobility (6 items), kitchen (5 items), domestic (5 items) and leisure (6 items). There are four response categories relating to achieving the item: 'on my own', 'on my own with difficulty', which both score 1; 'with help' and 'no', which both score 0. Total score ranges from 0–22; a high score indicates a more active individual.

The development of disease-specific ADL questionnaires is making this questionnaire one that is not likely to be first choice in the future. It is specifically an outcome measure and is currently being used in a large randomized, controlled trial that will report both short- and long-term benefits of rehabilitation. As yet, it should not be dismissed as not being useful as an outcome measure for pulmonary rehabilitation programmes for COPD patients until further investigation has been completed and published.

2: Canadian Occupational Performance Measure (COPM)

The COPM (Law et al. 1994) is now a widely used and accepted outcome measure for patients with chronic conditions. It is a generic measure designed to be used by occupational therapists to detect changes in functional performance and satisfaction over time. The patient identifies up to five problems in the areas of self-care, productivity and leisure using a 10-point scale of importance: 1 = not at all important and 10 = extremely important. Patients then rate their performance and satisfaction also using a 10-point scale: 1 = not able to do/not at all satisfied and 10 = able to do extremely well/extremely satisfied. On reassessment the same 10-point scales are used.

Scoring is carried out by separately summing the performance and satisfaction scores and dividing them by the number of problem areas. This provides mean scores for performance and satisfaction. A 2-point change in either direction after intervention indicates a clinically important change (Law et al. 1998).

It has been validated as a reliable tool in patients with COPD (Williams et al. 2001) and has also been found to be sensitive in detecting changes over time in patients with COPD (Williams et al. 2001, Mason et al. 1999).

Strength of the COPM is its strong link to OT theory, which is of importance to all practising occupational therapists. It is useful in problem identification, being very similar to the first part of the CRDQ (see Chapter 3) that identifies the five most important activities, with the degree of breathlessness experienced also rated with each activity. As a generic questionnaire, the COPM fails to address this particular factor that is so important to COPD patients. Although the COPM is valued for its contribution to assessment of interventions, it has also been considered as time-consuming and difficult to administer. Weight is placed upon the occupational therapist's interviewing skills and how they are able to encourage the patient to identify presenting problems. The COPM can be used as a guide to treatment, as well as an outcome measure.

(The following assessment specific to ADL has been used and is mentioned only for reference and future consideration.)

3: Functional Independence Measure (FIM)

In a recent study (Biscione et al. 2001), the FIM was used as an outcome measure. It concluded that in-patient pulmonary rehabilitation in elderly COPD patients improves not only exercise capacity but also other outcomes such as mobility, self-care, communication and social cognition. Use of the FIM in future studies is to be encouraged.

The development of a disease-specific ADL assessment by occupational therapists to assess OT intervention with COPD patients in pulmonary rehabilitation is an important future consideration. To the present day, the questionnaires available have been developed by disciplines other than OT and do not fully accord with the OT problem-based/client-centred philosophy and process. To raise the OT profile and develop the OT evidence base, this challenging project is a necessity.

References

Agle DP, Baum GL (1977) Psychological aspects of chronic obstructive pulmonary disease. Medical Clinics of North America 61(4): 749–58.

Agle DP, Baum GL, Chester EH, Wendt M (1973) Multidiscipline treatment of chronic pulmonary insufficiency: I. Psychologic aspects of rehabilitation. Psychosomatic Medicine 35(1): 41–49.

Ainsworth BE, Haskell WL, Leon AS et al. (1993) Compendium of Physical Activities: classification of energy costs of human activities. Medicine and Science in Sports and Exercise 25(1): 71–80.

Ainsworth BE, Haskell WL, Whitt MC et al. (2000) Compendium of Physical Activities: an update of activity codes and MET intensities. Med. Sci. Sports Exer. 32(9 Suppl): S498–S504.

Ando M, Mori A, Esaki H et al. (2003) The effect of pulmonary rehabilitation in patients with post-tuberculosis lung disorder. Chest 123(6): 1988–1995.

Anonymous (1997) Pulmonary rehabilitation: joint ACCP/AACVPR evidence-based guidelines. ACCP/AACVPR Pulmonary Rehabilitation Guidelines Panel. American College of Chest Physicians. American Association of Cardiovascular and Pulmonary Rehabilitation. Chest 112(5): 1363–1396.

Anonymous (2001) British Thoracic Society Standards of Care Subcommittee on Pulmonary Rehabilitation Pulmonary rehabilitation. Thorax 56: 827–834.

Bendstrup KE, Ingemann Jensen J, Holm S et al. (1997) Out-patient rehabilitation improves activities of daily living, quality of life and exercise tolerance in chronic obstructive pulmonary disease. European Respiratory Journal 10(12): 2801–2806.

Bernstein DA, Borkovec TD (1973) Progressive relaxation training: a manual for the helping professions. Champaign, Illinois: Research Press.

Bestall JC, Paul EA, Garrod R et al. (1999) Usefulness of the Medical Research Council (MRC) dyspnoea scale as a measure of disability in patients with chronic obstructive pulmonary disease. Thorax 54(7): 581–586.

Biscione GL, Dominici M, Fabiani F, Rossi S, Visconti G, Imperiali M, Pasqua F (2001) Efficacy of inpatient pulmonary rehabilitation in elderly COPD subjects (>70) using Functional Independence Measure (FIM). American Journal of Respiratory and Critical Care Medicine 163(5).

Bratton EC (1958) Some factors of cost to the body in standing or sitting to work under different postural conditions. Journal of Home Economics 50(9): 711–713.

Broussard R (1979) Using relaxation for COPD. American Journal of Nursing 79(11): 1962–1963.

Casaburi R, Petty TL (eds.) (1993) Principles and Practice of Pulmonary Rehabilitation. Philadelphia, Pa: WB Saunders & Company.

Cox T (1978) Stress. London: Macmillan.

Dempster OL, deRenne C (1985) Chronic Obstructive Pulmonary Disease: Program Guidelines for Occupational Therapists and other Health professionals. Ramsco Publishing Company.

ERS (1997) Task Force Position Paper. Selection criteria and programmes for pulmonary rehabilitation in COPD patients. European Respiratory Journal 10: 744–757.

Fontana D (1993) Managing Time. Leicester: British Psychological Society.

Gallefoss F, Bakke PS (1999) How does patient education and self-management among asthmatics and patients with chronic obstructive pulmonary disease affect medication? American Journal of Respiratory and Critical Care Medicine 160(6): 2000-2005.

Garrod R, Bestall JC, Paul EA et al. (2000) Development and validation of a standardized measure of activity of daily living in patients with severe COPD: the London Chest Activity of Daily Living scale (LCADL). Respiratory Medicine 94(6): 589–596.

Garrod R, Paul EA, Wedzicha JA (2002) An evaluation of the reliability and sensitivity of the London Chest ADL Scale (LCADL). Respiratory Medicine 96(9): 725–730.

Gift AG, Moore T, Soeken K (1992) Relaxation to reduce dyspnoea and anxiety in COPD. Nursing Research 41(4): 242–246.

Gilbert D (1965) Energy expenditures for the disabled homemaker, review of studies. American Journal of Occupational Therapy 19(6): 321–328.

Griffiths TL, Burr ML, Campbell IA et al. (2000) Results at 1 year of outpatient multidisciplinary pulmonary rehabilitation: a randomised controlled trial. Lancet 355(9201): 362–8.

Gunn SM, Brooks AG, Withers RT et al. (2002) Determining energy expenditure during some household and garden tasks. Medicine and Science in Sports and Exercise 34(5): 895–902.

Hodgkin JE, Zorn EG, Connors GL (eds.) (1984) Pulmonary Rehabilitation: Guidelines to Success. London: Butterworth.

Hodgkin JE, Zorn EG, Bell CW (eds.) (1993) Pulmonary Rehabilitation: Guidelines to Success (second edition). Philadelphia, Pa: Lippincott.

Jacobson E (1938) Progressive Relaxation (second edition). Chicago, Ill: The University of Chicago Press.

Jacobson E (1976) You Must Relax. London: Souvenir Press.

James S (2001) University of Wales College of Medicine. A study to investigate the validity and clinical utility of the Morriston OT Outcome Measure (MPhil dissertation).

Lareau SC, Carrieri-Kohlman V, Janson-Bjerklie S, Roos SJ (1994) Development and testing of the Pulmonary Functional Status and Dyspnea Questionnaire (PFSDQ). Heart and Lung: Journal of Acute and Critical Care 23(3): 242–250.

Lareau SC, Meek PM, Roos PJ (1998) Development and testing of the modified version of the pulmonary functional status and dyspnea questionnaire (PFSDQ-M). Heart and Lung: Journal of Acute and Critical Care 27(3): 159–168.

Larsen EM (1947) The fatigue of standing. American Journal of Physiology 150: 109–121.

Law M et al. (1994) Canadian Occupational Performance Measure (COPM). Ottawa, Ontario: Canadian Association of Occupational Therapists.

Law M, Baptiste S, Carswell A, McColl MA, Polatajko H, Pollock N (1998) Canadian Occupational Performance Measure (COPM) (third edition). Toronto, ON: CAOT Publications ACE.

Leidy N Kline, Knebel A (2000) The role of meaning, enjoyment and symptoms in the functional performance of patients with COPD. American Journal of Respiratory and Critical Care Medicine, Abstract, March, B82: A458.

Lichstein KL (1988) Clinical Relaxation Strategies. New York: John Wiley.

Lincoln NB, Gladman JR (1992) NEADL. Disability and Rehabilitation 14(1): 41–43.

Lincoln NB, Gladman JR (1993) NEADL. Age and Ageing 22: 419–424.

Madders J (1981) Stress and Relaxation: Self-help ways to cope with stress and relieve nervous tension, ulcers, insomnia, migraine and high blood pressure (third edition). London: Martin Dunitz.

Marcus BH, Owen N (1992) Motivational readiness, self-efficacy and decision-making for exercise. Journal of Applied Social Psychology 22: 3–16.

Mason L, Singh SJ, Morgan MDL (1999) Improvements in domestic function after pulmonary rehabilitation. BTS Thorax 54(Supplement 3) A17.

McCracken EC, Richardson M (1959) Human energy expenditures as criteria for design of household storage facilities. Journal of Home Economy 51: 198–206.

Mitchell L, Bartlett M (1987) Simple Relaxation: The Mitchell method of physiological relaxation for easing tension (second edition). London: Murray.

Morgan M and Singh S. (eds.) (1997) Practical Pulmonary Rehabilitation. London: Chapman & Hall Medical.

Niederman MS, Clemente PH, Fei AM, Feinsilver SH, Robinson DA, Ilowite JS, Bernstein MG (1991) Benefits of a multidisciplinary pulmonary rehabilitation programme. Improvements are independent of lung function. Chest 99(4): 798–804.

Nouri FM, Lincoln NB (1987) An extended ADL scale for stroke patients. Clinical Rehabilitation 1: 301–305.

Okubadejo AA, O'Shea L, Jones PW, Wedzicha JA (1997) Home assessment of activities of daily living in patients with severe chronic obstructive pulmonary disease on long-term oxygen therapy. European Respiratory Journal 10(7): 1572–1575.

Ostrow AC, Dzewaltowski DA (1985) Older adult's perception of physical activity based on age-role and sex-role appropriateness. Research Quarterly for Exercise and Sport 57(2): 167–169.

Paris HJ, Griffiths TL (2001) Recognition of anxiety and depression in patients referred to a pulmonary rehabilitation programme. American Journal of Respiratory and Critical Care Medicine, April.

Passmore R, Durnin JV (1955) Human Energy Expenditure. Physiol Review 35(4): 801–40.

Pulmonary Rehabilitation Course Booklet – Llandough Hospital, Wales. Revised (2001).

Renfroe KL (1988) Effect of progressive relaxation on dyspnoea and state of anxiety in patients with chronic obstructive pulmonary disease. Heart and Lung: the Journal of Critical Care 17(4): 408–413.

Restrick LJ, Paul EA, Braid GM, Cullinan P, Moore-Gillon J, Wedzicha JA (1993) Survey of activities of daily living in patients with severe COPD. Thorax 48: 936–46.

Sewell L, Singh SJ, Morgan MDL, Williams JE, Collier R (2001) Goal-directed therapy does not significantly improve outcomes in rehabilitation. American Journal of Respiratory and Critical Care Medicine 163(5): A13.

Singh SJ, Vora VA, Morgan MDL (1999) Does pulmonary rehabilitation benefit current and non-smokers? American Journal of Respiratory and Critical Care Medicine 159(3): A764.

Smoller JW, Pollack MH, Otto MW et al. (1996) Panic, anxiety, dyspnoea and respiratory disease. Theoretical and clinical considerations. American Journal of Respiratory and Critical Care Medicine 154(1): 6–17.

Walsh R (1986) Occupational therapy as part of a pulmonary rehabilitation program. Occupational Therapy Health Care 3(1): 65–77.

Wedzicha JA, Bestall JC, Garrod R et al. (1998) Randomized controlled trial of pulmonary rehabilitation in severe chronic obstructive pulmonary disease patients, stratified with the MRC dyspnoea scale. European Respiratory Journal 12(2): 363–369.

Williams JE, Singh SJ, Sewell L et al. (2001) Development of a self-reported Chronic Respiratory Questionnaire (CRQ-SR). Thorax 56(12): 954–959.

Withers NJ, Rudkin ST, White RJ (1999) Anxiety and Depression in severe chronic obstructive pulmonary disease: the effects of pulmonary rehabilitation. Journal of Cardiopulmonary Rehabilitation 19(6): 362–365.

Chapter 9
Physiotherapy and the management of dyspnoea

R. GARROD

Introduction

Earlier chapters in this book have described the principles of exercise training and appropriate programmes of physical exercise in greater detail. The exercise component, so crucial to effecting change in patients with respiratory disease, is generally prescribed and provided by the physiotherapist; however, other elements of the programme are often poorly described and may lack scientific evaluation. Physiotherapists have a historical position in the education of patients regarding breathing retraining and sputum-clearance techniques. This chapter explores, in more detail, the therapeutic management of dyspnoea along with newer adjuncts, such as the role of non-invasive ventilation, respiratory muscle training, transcutaneous neuromusculo-electrical stimulation and oxygen provision, all of which may be provided in conjunction with a training programme within the multidisciplinary collaboration.

Breathing retraining

Diaphragmatic breathing

Exercise dyspnoea, the predominant symptom associated with respiratory disease, has been defined as the 'perception, during muscular exercise, of the imbalance between the ventilatory demand and the ability of the chest-lung mechanics to fulfil this demand' (Guenard et al. 1995). Dyspnoea is a multi-factorial complex symptom, characterized by a loss of elastic recoil and airflow obstruction leading to hyperinflation and air trapping, which in turn places the respiratory muscles, in particular the diaphragm, in a position of reduced mechanical efficiency. Increased dyspnoea may be perceived as an inappropriate imbalance between length and tension of the muscles. The sense of effort contributing to dyspnoea is associated with the intensity and duration of work performed (Mahler et al. 1992).

138

Additionally, there is evidence that increased activity of the accessory muscles of breathing is associated with increased dyspnoea, while an increase in the activity of the diaphragm is associated with reduced dyspnoea (Breslin et al. 1990). This suggests that diaphragmatic breathing or abdominal breathing may be effective in reducing the sensation of dyspnoea in patients with respiratory disease. While this may be the case in patients with mild disease, it appears less effective in patients with severe chronic obstructive pulmonary disease (COPD) or where significant hyperinflation exists. In fact, authors have suggested that in severe COPD a breathing pattern of low volume may actually help to prevent muscle fatigue, although acting to the detriment of effective gas exchange (Begin and Grassino 1991).

One very early study showed improvements in ventilatory parameters such as increased tidal volume and improved arterial oxygen saturation with deep breathing (Sackner et al. 1974); however, later research suggests that this may be at the expense of an increased work of breathing. Gosselink et al. (1995) showed that, in patients with severe COPD, abdominal breathing caused increased abnormality of chest wall movement, increased dyspnoea, and a decrease in the mechanical efficiency of breathing. This work was confirmed by more recent authors who showed that, in a population of patients with severe COPD recovering from exacerbation, the effects of abdominal breathing were indeed negative (Vitacca et al. 1998). Improvements in arterial blood gases and saturation occurred at the expense of an increased work of breathing and increased dyspnoea. It may be hypothesized that the ability to improve arterial blood gases would be more beneficial during times of exacerbation or during exercise.

However, Gosselink et al. (1995) also compared the effect of abdominal breathing with normal breathing during loaded respiration (which would reflect breathing during exacerbation) and found similar negative effects. The effects of deep breathing are unknown for patients with reversible airway obstruction where hyperinflation is less; in these patients increases in arterial oxygen saturation may translate into improvements in dyspnoea and exercise tolerance. Since few studies incorporate subjective evaluation of patient preference, it is difficult to identify potential beneficiaries of deep breathing techniques or to know how to incorporate this information into a pulmonary rehabilitation programme.

Assessment of dyspnoea generally lacks sensitivity; we may know how breathless the patient perceives themselves to be using a validated measure such as the Borg Breathlessness Scale (Kendrick, et al. 2000), but do we actually speak the language of dyspnoea? Mahler and Harver (2000) discuss the use of descriptors of breathlessness and conclude that asking specific questions about the quality of breathlessness, the onset and precipitating factors could help us identify the cause of dyspnoea more accurately. To this end the authors have published a tool which may be useful in helping clinicians understand the context of breathlessness in greater depth (Harver et al. 2000). Feasibly, when a patient describes their breathlessness as 'breathing more', the use of slow controlled abdominal breathing may be helpful, whereas a patient who describes the perception as increased 'work and effort' may already be demonstrating signs of fatigue, in which case abdominal breathing will exacerbate this feeling. Furthermore, patients who complain of 'chest tightness' are describing an asthmatic component which might be better treated with medication, humidification and slow-breathing patterns.

Management of hyperventilation

The effect of concomitant hyperventilation syndrome in patients with respiratory disease is unknown and may be underestimated. There is evidence of associated hyperventilation in patients with asthma that will increase the sensation of dyspnoea; breathing education that focuses on deep breathing will exacerbate this condition, and measures should be employed to reduce the depth and frequency of breathing (Thomas et al. 2003). In a recent randomized, controlled trial, patients were taught diaphragmatic breathing in small groups for an initial 45 minutes and then two weeks later they received an individual review for 15 minutes. The control group received a 60-minute education session, again in small groups, from the respiratory nurse (Thomas et al. 2003). There was a significant difference between the groups, with the active group achieving an improvement in overall quality of life, and the change in the activities domain was still significant at six months. This is important work that should have application in pulmonary rehabilitation programmes when patients with asthma are included. Ideally, additional time should be provided in rehabilitation to allow for individual reinforcement of group learned techniques.

Buteyko Breathing Technique

The Buteyko Breathing Technique (BBT) has generated much interest in the past ten years. Originally from Russia, this breathing technique was designed to address problems of hyperventilation among patients with asthma. Although there has been much publicity concerning the technique, there remains a lack of evidence to support the technique. The one published study so far has a number of methodological flaws, particularly in the use of reduced medication therapy as a primary outcome measure (Bowler et al. 1998). Bowler et al. actively recruited patients who were high users of beta-2 agonists (>1400 mcg), and of 170 patients screened 77 per cent were excluded from the trial. The remaining 39 patients were randomized to a control group who received abdominal breathing, or an active group who received BBT and greater follow-up support. After three months, there were no differences in lung-function measures between the groups but there was a large and statistically significant difference in the usage of beta-2 agonists with the BBT. The groups were stratified for medication usage prior to randomization, with the active group reporting higher usage for both steroids and reliever medication at baseline. This method of stratification limits the strength of the evidence to support the technique. However, the authors observe that, in comparison with normal subjects, the asthma patients in both groups demonstrated a lower-end tidal CO_2 level; this suggests an element of hyperventilation was common to these patients. Like advocated physiotherapeutic management of hyperventilation (Thomas et al. 2003), the BBT method employs a breathing pattern to encourage slow frequency and reduced depth. Breath-holding techniques are encouraged within BBT, although the clinical efficacy of this has not been established. With the added complication of hyperventilation syndrome and/or dysfunctional breathing, the need for accurate assessment is reinforced. The use of a validated questionnaire, such as the Nijmegen Questionnaire (van Dixhoorn and Duivenvoorden 1985), to determine the prevalence of hyperventilation is advised.

A word of caution remains with the BBT, though: actively encouraging patients to reduce medication usage may be appropriate for patients who excessively use relievers through fear or panic, but the reduction of steroid and preventive medication may have deleterious effects on the control of asthma. Much larger trials are required before such an approach to medication advice could be advocated. Furthermore, adequate optimization of medication prior to pulmonary rehabilitation is recommended; according to British Thoracic Society steps for management, if patients are overly relying on short-term bronchodilators they should be referred back to the medical consultant for review (BTS 1997).

Relaxation techniques

It has been well documented that dyspnoea is associated with fear and helplessness (DeVito 1990, Smoller et al. 1996, O'Donnell 1994), and it is unsurprising that this 'dyspnoea spiral' is itself a cause of further disability. A proposed model, the cognitive-behavioural model, suggests that 'it is the individual's fear of and misinterpretation of the physical sensations associated with dyspnoea, hyperventilation, or other symptoms that are thought to be crucial in producing panic attacks' (Clark 1986). Recently, authors have used this model of panic in the development of a questionnaire to assess catastrophic cognitions (Gurney-Smith et al. 2002). Physiological relaxation techniques may be effective for patients where attacks are provoked or associated with a high degree of panic, in order to lower the heart rate and induce relaxation (Salt and Kerr 1997). Other relaxation techniques may be usefully taught as long as patients are able to incorporate them into their daily life rather than 'just at pulmonary rehabilitation'. Collaboration with other members of the multidisciplinary team will highlight the effectiveness of these interventions; liaison with clinical psychologists, home care respiratory nurses and occupational therapists can implement and reinforce good practice in the community.

Pursed-lips breathing

Many patients naturally adopt the use of pursed-lips breathing (PLB). This simple technique appears to have many physiological benefits in COPD. PLB has been identified as a potential mechanism for reducing dyspnoea during daily activities (Barach 1973), although it is unknown whether this enhances exercise tolerance. PLB involves the subject performing expiration through pursed lips, held in a whistling or kissing position, this creates increased resistance to expiration, which in turn reduces the flow of air during expiration. This enables the subject to breathe at a higher point on the lung pressure–volume curve (Ingram and Schilder 1967). For patients with COPD, PLB is associated with increased arterial saturation, beneficial changes in chest wall muscle recruitment and enhanced diaphragmatic activity (Breslin 1992). However, PLB may make the work of breathing harder since the subject is required to produce greater inspiratory pressures to initiate breathing. Additionally, abdominal muscle activity is increased during PLB, which may increase oxygen utilization. Indeed, Roa et al. showed in 12 subjects with COPD that, although PLB resulted in increases in tidal volume and reduction in respiratory rate, the overall work of breathing was greater than during tidal breathing (Roa et al. 1991). Much of the work concerning PLB is in abstract form only and predates 1975, making it difficult to form strong conclusions.

For patients who adopt the technique, naturally it would be inadvisable, and indeed impossible, to teach an alternative breathing pattern. However, the role of PLB in patients during exercise, when dynamic hyperinflation increases and the diaphragm is placed at greater mechanical disadvantage, is untested. Additionally, PLB in patients who do not adopt the technique naturally is unevaluated. Early data from our group suggest that in patients with COPD, naive to PLB, the use of this technique during exercise significantly lowers the post-exercise respiratory rate and improves time to recovery of baseline breathlessness. However, these benefits did not translate into increased walking distance or perception of end exercise dyspnoea. In the USA, PLB is routinely taught during functional activities as part of pulmonary rehabilitation, and although there are few published data, anecdotal evidence continues to support the use of this technique (Breslin 1995). Indeed, our early data suggest that benefits in terms of reduced respiratory rate are likely to be greatest in patients with resting breathlessness, and inappropriate for those without.

Positioning

The lean-forward sitting position has been shown to produce significant relief for a selection of patients with COPD; in particular, patients who demonstrate marked hyperinflation appear to show the greatest relief (Sharp et al. 1980). It has been suggested that the effect of the abdominal contents in lean-forward is to push the diaphragm into a position of greater mechanical efficiency by improving the length tension curve of the muscle fibres. This enhances the contraction of the diaphragm, while at the same time fixing the upper extremities and shoulder girdle appears to increase the effectiveness of the inspiratory accessory muscles. This was demonstrated by Sharp et al. by a reduction in electromyography of the accessory muscles with the lean-forward sitting position. The implications of this are clear: working in conjunction with occupational therapists, we can provide opportunities at home for effective positioning for the relief of dyspnoea. The provision of a chair at the top of stairs or a high shelf perhaps halfway up the stairs will enable a patient to climb stairs more easily, leaving energy for other activities. Home care team members from the outpatient pulmonary rehabilitation programme will be able to provide seamless integration into the community. While out walking, patients may be taught effective positions to adopt leaning against a wall, standing with hands fixed behind the back to fix the shoulder girdle or side leaning. Positions and management taught on the six- or eight-week programme must be translated into behaviour changes in the community; for this, all the team members need to be involved. Assessment of efficacy of therapy is required and may be performed simply with the aid of a breathing scale such as the visual analogue score (VAS) or the Borg Breathlessness Scale. The community team, often occupational therapy, physiotherapy, nursing and social work, need to be informed and included in the hospital process. One position may work better for one patient, one breathing technique be better for another; individualizing the therapy requires assessment and teamwork. Logistic problems may make this difficult; there will be resource implications, but where the effort to integrate the team is not made there will be overlap and redundancy, and the best treatment may get lost in the process.

Sputum clearance

While the aim of pulmonary rehabilitation is not primarily related to assisting sputum clearance, for patients with copious sputum it is likely that the exercise component contributes to improved efficacy. Data from patients with cystic fibrosis suggest that a 60-minute exercise component provided prior to traditional physiotherapeutic techniques significantly improves expectoration amounts (Baldwin et al. 1994).

Physiotherapeutic adjuncts to pulmonary rehabilitation

Having discussed the role of breathing exercise and positioning, it is worth considering the value of adjunctive treatments. Pulmonary rehabilitation is not effective for all patients. A study by Troosters et al. (2001) describes the potential characteristics of non-responders compared with responders. In their study, they found that patients with more severe ventilatory impairment and less respiratory and peripheral muscle weakness showed little benefit compared with patients with evidence of weakness and less severe impairment. Where lung impairment is so severe as to limit the intensity of training, other adjuncts may be usefully applied. In patients with severe COPD, respiratory muscle weakness and/or fatigue will contribute to dyspnoea during exhaustive exercise. Early studies suggest that the application of non-invasive positive pressure support during exercise reduces dyspnoea (Kyroussis et al. 1996) and delays diaphragmatic fatigue (Polkey et al. 1996).

Randomized controlled trials investigating the effect of non-invasive positive pressure ventilation (NIPPV) during exercise have shown improvements in exercise tolerance and reductions in dyspnoea (Bianchi et al. 1998, Keilty et al. 1994). The use of NIPPV during exercise enhances performance and improves dyspnoea, probably as a result of the unloading of the respiratory muscles. However, there are practical difficulties to providing ventilation during a training session, limiting the type of exercise and questioning the adherence to exercise. Moreover, there appears to be little effect of additional ventilatory support for patients with mild COPD (Bianchi et al. 2002).

Only one trial to date has evaluated the role of non-invasive ventilation provided nocturnally at home in conjunction with an outpatient rehabilitation programme (Garrod et al. 2000a). In this randomized controlled trial, there was a significant additional effect of ventilation on exercise tolerance (see Figure 9.1 below), health-related quality of life (see Figure 9.2 below) and arterial oxygenation. After four weeks of training, there were similar improvements in exercise tolerance in both groups; however, in the final four weeks of training, changes in the ventilation group became significantly greater, suggesting a dose response effect. Furthermore, only the group treated with non-invasive positive pressure ventilation showed improvement in inspiratory muscle strength, and the difference in the dyspnoea component of the CRDQ was clinically, although not statistically, different between the groups. Although for most patients exercise alone will be sufficient to achieve functional improvement, for more severely disabled patients, or those awaiting lung transplant surgery, the addition of NIPPV may augment benefits (Wedzicha and Beckles 2001). Physiotherapists will play a part in the assessment of patients appropriate for additional rehabilitation therapies. At present this is an early and relatively untested application of non-invasive ventilation; however, for patients who do not improve substantially with rehabilitation, other strategies may be required. Reassessment of these patients is required to identify the cause of non-response, and further stages should be implemented.

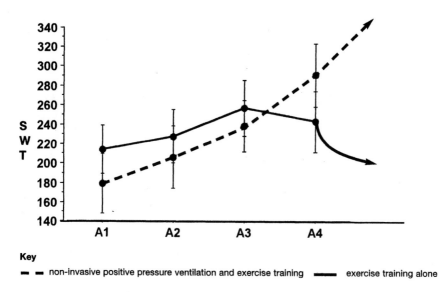

Figure 9.1 Repeated measures Analysis of Variance (ANOVA) showing change in SWT at each assessment (n = 30).

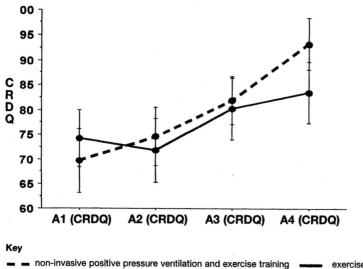

Figure 9.2 Repeated measures ANOVA showing change in CRDQ at each assessment (n = 30).

Neuromuscular electrical stimulation

A further adjunct to rehabilitation may include the use of neuromuscular electrical stimulation, particularly for patients too breathless to comply with an intensive programme or for patients who are unable to travel to outpatient rehabilitation programmes. A recent well-designed randomized controlled trial has shown a significant increase in exercise tolerance and peripheral muscle strength after a six-week home programme of neuromuscular electrical stimulation (NMES) to the quadriceps (Neder et al. 2000). Patients with severe COPD applied the technique at home after physiotherapy instruction and with weekly physiotherapy monitoring. The technique was well tolerated, and, along with physiological improvements, there was a reduction in perceived dyspnoea. This is an interesting development and may prove to have particular value for severely disabled housebound patients who respond poorly to aerobic training programmes (Wedzicha et al. 1998).

Respiratory muscle training and rehabilitation

For patients who demonstrate respiratory muscle weakness, respiratory muscle training may prove an appropriate adjunct to pulmonary rehabilitation. There have been conflicting reports concerning the additional effect of ventilatory muscle training (VMT) to general exercise. Wanke et al. (1994) showed an additional effect of VMT in COPD patients compared with cycle endurance alone, while other studies have shown no significant additive effects of VMT compared with general training alone (Berry et al. 1996, Larson et al. 1999). In a recent cross-over study, the cumulative effect of bronchodilators, exercise and VMT were studied (Weiner et al. 2000). The authors suggest that the addition of VMT was associated with an increase in respiratory muscle strength, whereas the addition of general exercise was associated with improvements in exercise tolerance. However, this study suffers from a number of methodological errors, making interpretation difficult. The same patients were randomized to different arms of the study a number of times, the control group that received bronchodilator plus general exercise plus sham VMT was small, with only five subjects, and there was no description of statistical analysis reported.

There is further contention concerning the effect of pulmonary rehabilitation on respiratory muscle performance in the absence of targeted respiratory muscle training. However, O'Donnell et al. (1998) demonstrated that, after six weeks of exercise training using maximal perceived breathlessness to target intensity, improvements in both peripheral and respiratory muscles were evident. Measurements were made using maximal inspiratory pressure (MIP), which may lack reliability due to voluntary effort. However, over a control period of six weeks, the same subjects showed no difference in MIP, suggesting that poor reliability was not a factor. Ries et al. (1995) have found no such changes in MIP with rehabilitation, which may relate to differences in the targeting of maximal intensity of training. It is feasible that, with sufficiently high-intensity general training, respiratory muscles will show similar adaptations to peripheral muscles due to increased respiratory effort with the physical training programme.

At present, respiratory muscle training as an adjunct to pulmonary rehabilitation is not routinely indicated. However, if a patient has undergone training and showed little response, assessment of maximal inspiratory and expiratory muscle strength may demonstrate an underlying weakness that has prevented effective training.

Supplemental oxygen and rehabilitation

Many patients are provided with cylinders of oxygen at home to be used for symptomatic relief as required; however, previous studies have shown variable results on the benefit of short-burst oxygen therapy. Patients report considerable symptomatic benefit and earlier recovery after exercise with short-burst oxygen therapy, though there is little evidence to support this finding, and effects may not be reproducible with time. There is a large degree of variability within patients in response to short-burst oxygen therapy, and predicting which patients will benefit is difficult (Evan et al. 1986). A recent publication has evaluated the role of short burst oxygen provided pre and post exercise in patients with severe COPD who demonstrated significant arterial desaturation. In this study there was little benefit of oxygen on dyspnoea, arterial saturation or exercise tolerance (Nandi et al. 2003). Contrary to scientific evidence, the majority of oxygen cylinders are prescribed for short-burst purposes, although individual daily usage is generally low (Okubadejo et al. 1994). These patients may become dependent on oxygen for symptomatic relief of dyspnoea, which in turn can limit activities and restrict daily life, particularly where no portable system is provided. This is important when considering the role of oxygen as part of pulmonary rehabilitation, since inappropriate provision may be more harmful than helpful.

Ambulatory oxygen, however, may play a more effective part in the management of patients with respiratory disease. A number of randomized trials have shown improvements in exercise tolerance while breathing supplemental oxygen (Woodcock et al. 1981, Garrod et al. 1999, Leggett and Flenley 1977) with the greatest improvements occurring during sub-maximal exercise (Bradley et al. 1978). Work investigating the mechanisms of improvement with supplemental oxygen show that there is a reduction in minute ventilation during exercise and that this reduction appears to be related to hypoxic drive (Stein et al. 1982, Woodcock et al. 1981). Lock et al. (1991) show a correlation between improvements in walking distance and arterial desaturation, indicating that ambulatory oxygen should be provided only where evidence of exercise desaturation exists. However, there is a large placebo effect on exercise while breathing oxygen, with Waterhouse and Howard (1983) showing an increase in walking on placebo (air cylinder) test that was equal to almost half of the increase resulting from oxygen. Individual assessments of the benefit of portable oxygen remain a requirement for ensuring efficacy.

Within the pulmonary rehabilitation team there will be a number of specialists trained to identify and establish oxygen requirements. The original medical consultation should highlight patients for whom long-term oxygen is indicated, but a baseline walking test will be required to identify those patients who demonstrate exercise desaturation (a drop of 4 per cent to below 90 per cent). This may be performed by any member of the team, and will be performed as part of the initial pulmonary rehabilitation assessment process. If arterial desaturation is identified, further assessment should be made to ensure adequate correction of oxygenation. For these patients, supplemental oxygen may be considered for pulmonary rehabilitation.

Studies have been published that attempt to establish whether supplemental oxygen enhances the effects of rehabilitation in these patients. (Rooyackers et al. 1997, Garrod, et al. 2000b). The results of both trials suggest that the additive effect of oxygen during rehabilitation is minimal. However, in the latter study there was a small but statistically significant effect of oxygen on dyspnoea, which was evident at the end of the training programme (Garrod et al. 2000b). Although the mechanisms for this are unknown, it is possible that reduced dyspnoea during training allayed anxiety and enabled patients to become further desensitized. A commentary on these two studies suggests that 'improvements in dyspnoea alone may make it worth applying supplemental oxygen during training programmes in COPD patients' (Yilmaz 2001). It is important to remember that, where oxygen is provided for the training programme, it should also be encouraged for community use. The message is ambiguous if oxygen is provided only for the purpose of the rehabilitation programme, and, in these cases, adherence to the home exercise programme may be compromised. Respiratory nurses, occupational therapists and community physiotherapists will be instrumental in ensuring that adequate provision is made in the community. A pragmatic approach is required where there is no facility for home-portable oxygen or where patients refuse to use ambulatory systems. It is perhaps reassuring to note that, even though significant falls in arterial desaturation have been documented in pulmonary rehabilitation programmes, there were no ill effects in patients who exercised with placebo air (Garrod et al. 2000b).

Mobility

Patients entered into pulmonary rehabilitation programmes may have problems other than those caused by respiratory disease, and other musculoskeletal problems are common in older patients. Likely problems can include a range of conditions from osteoarthritis of the lumbar and sacral region to joint-replacement surgery. Ultimately, the role of the physiotherapist within the pulmonary rehabilitation team will be to assess the patient and determine fitness for training and make any adaptations to exercise that may be relevant.

It is important to pay attention to the home environment and ensure that exercises that are applicable within the hospital setting can be translated into home training programmes. Where positions are adapted because of pain, the community team will need to check that this can be carried out in a similar manner at home in order to avoid damaging exercise when the patient is independent. For patients with kyphotic and scoliotic postures, there may be particular problems with thoracic joint stiffness, and a treatment of exercises aimed specifically at mobilizing the thorax may be useful. The common 'barrel chest' abnormality will lead to reduced mobility of the sternum, rib cage and rib attachments. Excessive accessory muscle use often leads to tension in the shoulder girdle and the cervical region; both areas may benefit from deep massage techniques. Physiotherapists may also be instrumental in providing walking aids where necessary; high rolators that enable patients to fix the shoulder girdle are often beneficial for patients, particularly when ambulatory oxygen is used in order to support the weight of the equipment. A walking stick with a folding seat may be used to enable rest periods during mobilization. Where patients are prescribed walking aids, any walking tests performed should be carried out using the aid. Table 9.1 provides an evaluation of the possible causes of dyspnoea and suggested physiotherapeutic treatments.

To carry out a full and adequate assessment of the pulmonary patient will take time, and to be inclusive and comprehensive all members of the multidisciplinary team should be involved. Spirometry and lung-function assessment will be carried out by a respiratory technician, assessment and identification of learning needs may be carried out by respiratory nurse, while activities of daily living and physical mobility and strength will be carried out by occupational therapists and physiotherapists. Utilizing all the team members ensures a thorough and inclusive assessment procedure. Assessment time should be allocated and incorporated into the original budgeting of the rehabilitation programme; without accurate assessment, the rehabilitation process will lack effectiveness.

Table 9.1 Approaches to different causes of dyspnoea

Possible cause of dyspnoea in COPD	Possible treatment
Hyperinflation	PLB/positioning
Hypoxia	Ambulatory oxygen therapy / LTOT
Peripheral muscle fatigue	Peripheral muscle training, neuromuscular electrical stimulation
Hyperventilation	Slow frequency, reduced depth, breath holding
Postural dysfunction	Thoracic mobilization
Bronchoconstriction	Teach effective use of medications/Ensure optimization of medical (Asthma/COPD steps for treatment)
Panic/anxiety	Relaxation techniques, diaphragmatic breathing, cognitive-behavioural approach
Respiratory muscle fatigue	Non-invasive ventilation, positioning/Intermittent Positive Pressure Breathing
Sputum retention	Bronchopulmonary hygiene techniques
Respiratory muscle weakness	Respiratory muscle training

References

Baldwin DR, Hill AL, Peckham DG et al. (1994) Effect of addition of exercise to chest physiotherapy on sputum expectoration and lung function in adults with cystic fibrosis. Respiratory Management 88(1): 49–53.

Barach AL (1973) Physiologic advantages of grunting, groaning, and pursed-lip breathing: adaptive symptoms related to the development of continuous positive pressure breathing. Bulletin of the New York Academy of Medicine 49(8): 666–673.

Begin P, Grassino A (1991) Respiratory muscle dysfunction and chronic hypercapnia in chronic obstructive pulmonary disease. American Review of Respiratory Disease 143: 905–912.

Berry MJ, Adair NE, Sevensky KS et al. (1996) Inspiratory muscle training and whole-body reconditioning in chronic obstructive pulmonary disease. American Journal of Respiratory and Critical Care Medicine 153 (6 part 1): 1812–1816.

Bianchi L, Foglio K, Pagani M et al. (1998) Effects of proportional assist ventilation on exercise tolerance in COPD patients with chronic hypercapnia. European Respiratory Journal 11(2): 422–427.

Bianchi L, Foglio K, Porta R et al. (2002) Lack of additional effect of adjunct of assisted ventilation to pulmonary rehabilitation in mild COPD patients. Respiratory Management 96(5): 359–367.

Bowler SD, Green A, Mitchell CA (1998) Buteyko breathing techniques in asthma: a blinded randomised controlled trial. Medical Journal of Australia 169(11–12): 575–578.

Bradley BL, Garner AE, Billiu D et al. (1978) Oxygen-assisted exercise in chronic obstructive lung disease. The effect on exercise capacity and arterial blood gas tensions. American Review of Respiratory Disease 118(2): 239–243.

Breslin EH (1992) The pattern of respiratory muscle recruitment during pursed-lip breathing. Chest 101(1): 75–78.

Breslin EH (1995) Breathing retraining in chronic obstructive pulmonary disease. Journal of Cardiopulmonary Rehabilitation 15(1): 25–33.

Breslin EH, Garoutte BC, Kohlman-Carrieri V et al. (1990) Correlations between dyspnea, diaphragm and sternomastoid recruitment during inspiratory resistance breathing in normal subjects. Chest 98(2): 298–302.

British Thoracic Society (BTS) (1997) Standards of Care Committee. Guidelines on the management of COPD. Thorax 52(Supplement 5): S1–S32.

Clark DM (1986) A cognitive approach to panic. Behaviour Research and Therapy 24:461-470.

DeVito AJ (1990) Dyspnea during hospitalizations for acute phase of illness as recalled by patients with chronic obstructive pulmonary disease. Heart and Lung: the Journal of Critical Care 19(2): 186–191.

Evan TW, Waterhouse JC, Carter A et al. (1986) Short burst oxygen treatment for breathlessness in chronic obstructive airways disease. Thorax 41: 611–615.

Garrod R, Bestall JC, Paul E et al. (1999) Evaluation of pulsed dose oxygen delivery during exercise in patients with severe chronic obstructive pulmonary disease. Thorax 54(3): 242–244.

Garrod R, Mikelsons C, Paul EA et al. (2000a) Randomized controlled trial of domiciliary non-invasive positive pressure ventilation and physical training in severe chronic obstructive pulmonary disease. American Journal of Respiratory and Critical Care Medicine 162(4 part 1): 1335–1341.

Garrod R, Paul EA, Wedzicha JA (2000b) Supplemental oxygen during pulmonary rehabilitation in patients with COPD with exercise hypoxaemia. Thorax 55(7): 539–543.

Gosselink RA, Wagenaar RC, Rijswijk H et al. (1995) Diaphragmatic breathing reduces efficiency of breathing in patients with chronic obstructive pulmonary disease. American Journal of Respiratory and Critical Care Medicine 151(4): 1136–1142.

Guenard H, Gallego J, Dromer C (1995) Exercise dyspnoea in patients with respiratory disease. European Respiratory Review 25: 6–13.

Gurney-Smith B, Cooper MJ, Wallace LM (2002) Anxiety and panic in chronic obstructive pulmonary disease: the role of catastrophic thoughts. Cognitive Therapy and Research 26(1): 143–155.

Harver A, Mahler DA, Schwartzstein RM et al. (2000) Descriptors of breathlessness in healthy individuals: distinct and separable constructs. Chest 118(3): 679–690.

Ingram RH Jr., Schilder DP (1967) Effect of pursed lips expiration on the pulmonary pressure-flow relationship in obstructive lung disease. American Review of Respiratory Disease 96(3): 381–388.

Keilty SE, Ponte J, Fleming TA et al. (1994) Effect of inspiratory pressure support on exercise tolerance and breathlessness in patients with severe stable chronic obstructive pulmonary disease. Thorax 49(10): 990–994.

Kendrick KR, Baxi SC, Smith RM (2000) Usefulness of the modified 0-10 Borg scale in assessing the degree of dyspnea in patients with COPD and asthma. Journal of Emergency Nursing 26(3): 216–222.

Kyroussis D, Polkey MI, Keilty SE et al. (1996) Exhaustive exercise slows inspiratory muscle relaxation rate in chronic obstructive pulmonary disease. American Journal of Respiratory and Critical Care Medicine 153(2): 787–793.

Larson JL, Covey MK, Wirtz SE et al. (1999) Cycle ergometer and inspiratory muscle training in chronic obstructive pulmonary disease. American Journal of Respiratory and Critical Care Medicine 160(2): 500–507.

Leggett RJ, Flenley DC (1977) Portable oxygen and exercise tolerance in patients with chronic hypoxic cor pulmonale. British Medical Journal 2(6079): 84–86.

Lock SH, Paul EA, Rudd RM et al. (1991) Portable oxygen therapy: assessment and usage. Respiratory Management 85(5): 407–412.

Mahler DA, Faryniarz K, Tomlinson D et al. (1992) Impact of dyspnea and physiologic function on general health status in patients with chronic obstructive pulmonary disease. Chest 102(2): 395–401.

Mahler DA, Harver A (2000) Do you speak the language of dyspnea? Chest 117(4): 928–929.

Nandi K, Smith AA, Crawford A et al. (2003) Oxygen supplementation before or after submaximal exercise in patients with chronic obstructive pulmonary disease. Thorax 58(8): 670–673.

Neder JA, Jones PW, Nery LE et al. (2000) Determinants of the exercise endurance capacity in patients with chronic obstructive pulmonary disease. The power–duration relationship. American Journal of Respiratory and Critical Care Medicine 162(2 part 1): 497–504.

O'Donnell DE (1994) Breathlessness in patients with chronic airflow limitation. Mechanisms and management. Chest 106(3): 904–912.

O'Donnell DE, McGuire M, Samis L et al. (1998) General exercise training improves ventilatory and peripheral muscle strength and endurance in chronic airflow limitation. American Journal of Respiratory and Critical Care Medicine 157(5 part 1): 1489–1497.

Okubadejo AA, Paul EA, Wedzicha JA (1994) Domiciliary oxygen cylinders: indications, prescription and usage. Respiratory Management 88(10): 777–785.

Polkey MI, Kyroussis D, Mills GH et al. (1996) Inspiratory pressure support reduces slowing of inspiratory muscle relaxation rate during exhaustive treadmill walking in severe COPD. American Journal of Respiratory and Critical Care Medicine 154(4 part 1): 1146–1150.

Ries AL, Kaplan RM, Limberg TM et al. (1995) Effects of pulmonary rehabilitation on physiologic and psychosocial outcomes in patients with chronic obstructive pulmonary disease. Annals of Internal Medicine 122(11): 823–832.

Roa J, Epstein S, Breslin EH et al. (1991) Work of breathing and ventilatory muscle recruitment during PLB in patients with chronic airway obstruction (abstract). American Review of Respiratory Disease 143: A77.

Rooyackers JM, Dekhuijzen PN, Van Herwaarden CL et al. (1997) Training with supplemental oxygen in patients with COPD and hypoxaemia at peak exercise. European Respiratory Journal 10(6): 1278–1284.

Sackner MA, Silva G, Banks JM et al. (1974) Distribution of ventilation during diaphragmatic breathing in obstructive lung disease. American Review of Respiratory Disease 109(3): 331–337.

Salt V, Kerr K (1997) Mitchell's Simple Physiological Relaxation and Jacobson's Progressive Relaxation Techniques: a comparison. Physiotherapy 83(4): 200–204.

Sharp JT, Drutz WS, Moisan T et al. (1980) Postural relief of dyspnea in severe chronic obstructive pulmonary disease. American Review of Respiratory Disease 122(2): 201–211.

Smoller JW, Pollack MH, Otto MW et al. (1996) Panic anxiety, dyspnea, and respiratory disease. Theoretical and clinical considerations. American Journal of Respiratory and Critical Care Medicine 154(1): 6–17.

Stein DA, Bradley BL, Miller WC (1982) Mechanisms of oxygen effects on exercise in patients with chronic obstructive pulmonary disease. Chest 81(1): 6–10.

Thomas M, McKinley RK, Freeman E et al. (2003) Breathing retraining for dysfunctional breathing in asthma: a randomised controlled trial. Thorax 58(2): 110–115.

Troosters T, Gosselink R, Decramer M (2001) Exercise training in COPD: how to distinguish responders from non-responders. Journal of Cardiopulmonary Rehabilitation 21(1): 10–17.

van Dixhoorn J, Duivenvoorden HJ (1985) Efficacy of Nijmegen Questionnaire in recognition of the hyperventilation syndrome. Journal of Psychosomatic Research 29(2): 199–206.

Vitacca M, Clini E, Bianchi L et al. (1998) Acute effects of deep diaphragmatic breathing in COPD patients with chronic respiratory insufficiency. European Respiratory Journal 11(2): 408–415.

Wanke T, Formanek D, Lahrmann H et al. (1994) Effects of combined inspiratory muscle and cycle ergometer training on exercise performance in patients with COPD. European Respiratory Journal 7(12): 2205–2211.

Waterhouse JC, Howard P (1983) Breathlessness and portable oxygen in chronic obstructive airways disease. Thorax 38(4): 302–306.

Wedzicha JA, Beckles M (2001) Non-invasive ventilation and pulmonary rehabilitation. European Respiratory Monograph 6(16): 238–243.

Wedzicha JA, Bestall JC, Garrod R et al. (1998) Randomized controlled trial of pulmonary rehabilitation in severe chronic obstructive pulmonary disease patients, stratified with the MRC dyspnoea scale. European Respiratory Journal 12(2): 363–369.

Weiner P, Magadle R, Berar-Yanay N et al. (2000) The cumulative effect of long-acting bronchodilators, exercise, and inspiratory muscle training on the perception of dyspnea in patients with advanced COPD. Chest 118(3): 672–678.

Woodcock AA, Gross ER, Geddes DM (1981) Oxygen relieves breathlessness in 'pink puffers'. Lancet 1(8226): 907–909.

Yilmaz GK (2001) Supplemental oxygen during training in COPD. European Respiratory Topics 7: 24–25.

Chapter 10
Dietary management of COPD

E. WOUTERS, A. SCHOLS, M. VERMEEREN

Introduction

Weight loss is a phenomenon that has long been recognized in the clinical course of chronic obstructive pulmonary disease (COPD) patients. Fowler and Godlee (1898) first described this association in patients with emphysema in the late nineteenth century. Attempts to describe different COPD classifications retained body weight as an important discriminator (Dornhurst 1955, Filley et al. 1968). In the 1960s, several studies reported that a low body weight and weight loss are negative predictive factors of survival in COPD (Vandenbergh et al. 1967). At that time, weight loss was considered to be an integral part of the clinical picture of chronic bronchitis; without adequate analysis of the underlying mechanisms or related functional consequences, nutritional depletion was considered an inevitable and irreversible terminal event related to the severity of airflow obstruction. It was even hypothesized that weight loss could be considered an adaptive mechanism in order to decrease oxygen consumption.

Although the importance of nutrition in health and disease is intuitively acknowledged, attention to the implications of weight loss on morbidity and mortality has only gained interest during the past decades. Later studies have demonstrated that low body mass index (BMI: weight divided by height in m^2) is a prognostic factor in COPD independent of the degree of airflow obstruction (Wilson et al. 1989, Landbo et al. 1999). In the same period, it became clear that muscle weakness has an important negative effect on morbidity in COPD patients, focusing attention on the pathophysiological implications of nutritional depletion. Recent data also demonstrated that being underweight is an independent risk factor for the development of COPD during life (Harik-Khan et al. 2002). Based on these observations, dietary management has to be considered as an important part of the disease management in patients suffering from COPD.

Assessment of nutritional status

Patients suffering from a chronic wasting disease like COPD are generally characterized by low body weight or loss of body weight. Body weight must be measured in a standardized setting using a calibrated scale with the patients barefoot and in light clothing. Body height has to be measured with a stadiometer with patients standing upright without wearing shoes.

Patients are considered underweight if they have a body weight less than 90 per cent of their ideal weight, based on the 1983 Metropolitan Life Insurance tables (Anonymous 1983). Characterization of nutritional depletion by percentage of ideal body weight, however, does not consider differences in body composition among individuals. The assessment of body composition has gained recent interest, since new indirect techniques have become available to estimate several different body compartments accurately with no discomfort for the investigated subjects. The most well-known body composition model is a two-compartment model, which divides the body into fat mass compartment (FMC) and the fat free mass (FFM). FFM can be further subdivided into two compartments: the intracellular compartment (also known as body cell mass or BCM), which represents the energy exchanging part, and the extracellular compartment, which represents substances outside the cells (such as collagen, fascia, plasma and interstitial fluid) and mainly functions as support and transport tissue. BCM reflects the quantity of actively metabolizing (liver, gut and immune system) and contracting (muscle) tissue. Approximately 60 per cent of the BCM is composed of muscle tissue. Since there is no method to measure BCM clinically, it is generally acknowledged that a useful estimate is given by the FFM. In relation to the pathophysiological implications of depletion, body composition analysis seems appropriate when conducted under stable conditions (Schols et al. 1991a).

Different methods are available to assess FFM. Anthropometric data, which can be obtained easily, consist of body height, weight, skinfold thickness and arm circumference. The biceps, triceps, subscapular and suprailiac sites are the generally selected skinfolds and can be measured by a specially designed analyser. One of the most well-known equations for measurement of FMC was developed by Durnin and Womersley (1974) and is based on the logarithmic transformation of the sum of four skinfold thicknesses, age and gender.

The precision of a skinfold thickness measurement is dependent upon the skill of the investigator and the site of measurement. On the basis of the measurement of midarm circumference (MAC) and triceps skinfold thickness, equations have also been developed to predict arm muscle area (AMA).

During recent years, bioelectrical impedance analysis (BIA) has been proposed as a quick, easy and reliable technique for the assessment of body composition. Impedance methods rely upon the differences in electrical conductivity of FFM and FMC. Body fluids, containing electrolytes, are, in general, responsible for the electrical conduction (reciprocal of resistance – R), while cell membranes determine the capacitance of the body (C). The reciprocal of C is equivalent to a resistance for an alternating current and is indicated by the impedance of capacitance. When inductance of the system can be neglected, capacitance is the main determining factor of the reactance of the system, X. For the alternating electrical current uses (800 μA, 50 kHz), the impedance (Z) will be determined by the R and reactance (X) in series according to the formula $Z = 0.5(R^2+X^2)$ (Lukaski et al. 1985). Z is related to the conductor length, the cross-sectional area of the conductor and signal frequency. BIA can easily be measured by applying electrodes on the dorsal site of the foot and hand with the patient in a supine position.

Calculation of FFM relies on the assumption of a constant ratio between total body water and FFM of 0.73. BIA has proved to be a reliable (Schols et al. 1991b) and reproducible (Schols et al. 1990) technique for the assessment of FFM in stable COPD patients, while anthropometry leads to significant overestimation of FFM, particularly in elderly patients.

FFM can be considered as a good estimate of BCM only when excessive fluid shifts between intracellular (ICW) and extracellular (ECW) water compartments are absent. Indeed, in acute wasting conditions or after a catabolic stress, the BCM can be decreased, whereas the ECW is absolutely or relatively expanded. It was found that in stable COPD patients the ratio between ECW and ICW is relatively constant. However, in patients with extreme wasting of FFM an increase in the ECW/ICW ratio was found (Baarends et al. 1997a).

At present, bioelectrical impedance can be assessed at one frequency (50 kHz) or using a spectrum of 48 frequencies ranging from 5 to 500 kHz. It was demonstrated that this bioelectrical impedance spectroscopy was not superior to BIA at 50 kHz to predict actual total body water (TBW) in stable COPD patients (Baarends et al. 1998a).

The importance of body composition analysis was demonstrated in studies characterizing large groups of clinically stable COPD patients. It was found that COPD patients can be stratified into four groups, based on a two-compartmental model:

- COPD patients with normal weight and normal FFM
- underweight patients and depletion of FFM
- underweight patients with preservation of FFM
- normal weight patients but with depletion of FFM (Engelen et al. 1994, Schols et al. 1993).

Biochemically, depletion of FFM is significantly related to the creatinine height index, as calculated by dividing the 24-hour urinary creatinine excretion of the patient by a reference value based on ideal body weight

(Schols et al. 1993). The index has received widespread clinical acceptance as a biochemical indicator of muscle mass. Hepatic secretory proteins such as albumin, pre-albumin, transferrin or retinol binding protein are often considered as indicators of visceral protein stores in comprehensive nutritional assessment programmes. However, these parameters reflect the inflammatory state of the patient and can definitely not be considered as indicators of nutritional state (Soeters et al. 1990, Tuten et al. 1985).

Recently, dual-energy x-ray absorptiometry (DXA) was introduced to differentiate body composition into three compartments. DXA directly assesses bone mineral content (Mazess et al. 1990) and the soft tissue surrounding the bone (Mazess et al. 1990, Lukaski 1987) by measuring the amount of fat and lean tissue. For that purpose, it is commonly used for accurate estimation of fat, bone and bone-free lean mass (Mazess et al. 1990, Jensen et al. 1993, Haarbo et al. 1991). Also, bone mineral density (BMD) (bone mineral content normalized for bone size) of the whole body and subregional compartments can be assessed. Because DXA is accepted as a safe, convenient and non-invasive method, it is well applicable in clinical practice as well as in the elderly, especially because the results are immediately available. Engelen et al. (1998) have clearly demonstrated that this method is valid in specific patient populations in COPD. Furthermore, DXA allows determination of patterns of tissue depletion; in particular, wasting of extremity FFM in COPD patients is reported to be associated with skeletal muscle weakness, independent of airflow obstruction (Engelen et al. 2000).

Energy balance in COPD

Weight loss occurs if energy expenditure exceeds dietary intake. Therefore, weight loss in patients with COPD may be caused by altered energy and substrate metabolism (hypermetabolism) or reduced dietary intake. More specifically, muscle wasting is a consequence of an imbalance between protein synthesis and protein breakdown. Impairments in total energy balance and protein metabolism may occur simultaneously, but these processes can also be dissociated because of altered regulation of substrate metabolism.

Altered energy and substrate metabolism in COPD

Total daily energy expenditure (TDE) is usually divided into three components:

1. resting energy expenditure (REE), comprising sleeping metabolic rate and the energy cost of arousal
2. diet-induced thermogenesis
3. physical-activity-induced thermogenesis.

By gas exchange measurement of patients in awake, relaxed conditions after an overnight fast, it is now possible to measure REE conveniently. Under these conditions, the thermic effect of food is considered insignificant, and it is assumed that the ambient temperature is within the thermoneutral zone for the individual. Based on the assumption that REE is the major component of total energy expenditure in sedentary persons, several studies have measured REE in COPD. REE was found to be elevated in 25 per cent of patients with COPD after adjustment for the metabolically active FFM (Creutzberg et al. 1998a). Whereas in healthy control subjects the amount of FFM explained up to 84 per cent of the individual variation in REE, it explained only 43 per cent in patients with COPD. Thus, other factors, such as work of breathing, drug therapy and systemic inflammation, may explain intersubject variability in REE. For example, a likely cause of the increased resting metabolic rate in patients with COPD is increased respiratory muscle work, given that the energy cost of ventilation is higher in patients with advanced disease than in healthy controls of comparable age and gender. Studies investigating this issue, however, have demonstrated conflicting results. Some studies have shown a relationship between REE and oxygen cost of ventilation (Jounieaux and Mayeux 1995, Mannix et al. 1992), whereas others have not (Baarends et al. 1998a, Sridhar et al. 1994). Part of this controversy can be explained by methodological pitfalls, such as variability in the technique to measure the oxygen cost of ventilation and inappropriate adjustment of REE for the metabolically active tissue mass. These factors were eliminated in a study (Hugli et al. 1995) comparing REE before and after nasal intermittent positive pressure ventilation (NIPPV) that eliminates diaphragmatic and intercostal activity. If elevated, REE was attributable to increased respiratory muscle work, and a demonstration of a reduction in REE might be expected following a period of respiratory muscle rest. No reduction in REE was observed, however, in a group of hypermetabolic patients after NIPPV (Hugli et al. 1995).

Beta-2 agonists are used commonly as maintenance bronchodilator therapy in patients with COPD, and the question has been raised as to whether beta-2 agonists might be responsible for the elevation noted in REE. Two weeks of salbutamol increased REE by less than 8 per cent in healthy males (Wilson et al. 1993). Acute inhalations of clinical doses of salbutamol, on the other hand, have been shown to increase REE by up to 20 per cent in healthy subjects in a dose-dependent manner (Amoroso et al. 1993). High doses of nebulized salbutamol are commonly administered during acute disease exacerbations. Nevertheless, no significant acute metabolic effect of this treatment was shown in elderly patients with COPD in comparison with an age-matched control group (Creutzberg et al. 1998b). Thus, bronchodilator therapy does not clearly account for elevations of REE in these patients.

Another factor contributing to hypermetabolism may be augmented to systemic inflammation. Tumour necrosing factor alpha (TNF-α) is a pro-inflammatory mediator produced by different cell types. It also triggers the release of other cytokines that mediate an increase in energy expenditure, as well as mobilization of amino acids and muscle protein catabolism. Using different markers, several studies have provided clear evidence for involvement of TNF-α related systemic inflammation in the pathogenesis of tissue depletion. Elevated levels of TNF-α (de Godoy et al. 1996, Francia et al. 1994) in plasma and in soluble TNF-receptors (Schols et al. 1996) were found in patients with COPD, particularly those suffering from weight loss. Some studies have shown a direct relationship between TNF-α levels and resting metabolic rate (Nguyen et al. 1999), whereas others have reported an association between REE and elevated levels of acute-phase proteins (Schols et al. 1996). In one study, hypermetabolic patients with an acute-phase response had a significantly lower FFM than hypermetabolic patients without the acute-phase reaction, despite a comparable BMI (Schols et al. 1996). These results indicate that systemic inflammation may cause hypermetabolism and induce a catabolic response.

In a subsequent study, such a relationship was demonstrated among the acute-phase protein lipopolysaccharide-binding protein, REE and decreased plasma amino acid levels used as a global marker of altered protein metabolism (Pouw et al. 1998).

Despite the methodologic difficulties in measuring TDE, recent studies have focused attention on activity-related energy expenditure in patients with COPD. Using the doubly labelled water ($^2H_2O^{18}$) technique to measure TDE, it was demonstrated that patients with COPD also had a significantly higher TDE than healthy subjects (Baarends et al. 1997b). Remarkably, the non-resting component of TDE was significantly higher in the patients with COPD than in the healthy subjects, resulting in a ratio between TDE and REE of 1.7 in patients with COPD and 1.4 in healthy subjects. Otherwise, when TDE was measured in patients with COPD and healthy persons in a respiration chamber, no difference in TDE was found between patients with COPD and healthy persons (Hugli 1996), possibly because of limitations of activities in the respiration chamber.

Several processes may account for the increased activity-related energy expenditure in patients with COPD. The mechanical efficiency of leg exercise is decreased in patients with COPD (Baarends et al. 1997b). Clearly, part of the increased oxygen consumption during exercise can also be related to inefficient ventilation in the presence of increased ventilatory demand, especially under conditions of dynamic hyperinflation (Baarends et al. 1997c). Furthermore, inefficient muscle metabolism may contribute to an increased TDE metabolism. Several studies showed severely impaired oxidative phosphorylation during exercise in COPD, accompanied by an increased and highly anaerobic metabolism involving both the energy release from high-energy phosphate compounds as well as enhanced glycolysis (Wuyam et al. 1992). It is generally known that anaerobic metabolism is less efficient than aerobic metabolism.

Therefore, the more active patients are especially at risk of an energy imbalance (Goris et al. 2003).

The fact that no difference in TDE was found between hypermetabolic and normometabolic patients with COPD, and that REE adjusted for FFM did not correlate significantly with TDE, indicates that different mechanisms may underlie metabolic alterations in subgroups of patients with COPD (Schols 1999).

Reduced dietary intake

Hypermetabolism can explain why some patients with COPD lose weight despite an apparently normal to even high dietary intake (Hunter et al. 1981). Nevertheless, it has been shown that dietary intake in weight-losing patients is lower than in weight-stable patients, both in absolute terms and in relation to measured REE (Schols et al. 1991c). This finding is quite remarkable because the normal adaptation to an increase in energy requirements in healthy men is an increase in dietary intake. The reasons for a relatively low dietary intake in COPD are not completely understood. It has been suggested that patients with COPD eat suboptimally because chewing and swallowing alter breathing patterns and lead to decreased arterial oxygen saturation. Although in one study no changes in arterial oxygen saturation (SaO_2) were observed in normoxemic patients with COPD during a meal (Schols et al. 1991d), hypoxemic patients experienced a rapid decrease in SaO_2 that recovered slowly after completion of the meal (Schols et al. 1991d). The decrease in SaO_2 was associated with an increased dyspnoea sensation. The severity of the drop was significantly different between two meals, but it could not be determined from the study whether this difference related to the macronutrient composition of the meal (less desaturation after a carbohydrate-rich meal) or meal temperature (more desaturation after a warm meal). The gastric emptying time of a meal may also affect dietary intake because gastric filling in these patients may limit diaphragm excursion, reduce the functional residual capacity, and lead to an increase in dyspnoea (Akrabawi et al. 1996). In addition to these effects of eating on the respiratory system, systemic factors may also affect dietary intake. Recent studies point towards the existence of altered regulation of appetite, possibly mediated by systemic inflammation. The adipocyte-derived hormone leptin is the afferent hormonal signal to the brain in a feedback mechanism that regulates fat mass. Circulating leptin levels correlate with BMI and fat percentage in healthy subjects. A similar observation was found in patients with COPD (Takabatake et al. 1999), but in some patients leptin levels were increased when adjusted for fat mass (Schols et al. 1999). A significant correlation was found between adjusted leptin levels and levels of soluble TNF-receptors (TNF55) (as marker of systemic inflammation) particularly in patients of the emphysematous subtype (Schols et al. 1999). Leptin levels, as well as soluble TNF55 levels in turn, were inversely related to dietary intake adjusted for REE. These data are consistent with experimental animal studies showing that administration of endotoxins or cytokines produced a prompt increase in serum leptin levels (Grunfeld et al. 1996) and a decrease in appetite and dietary intake. Temporary disturbances in energy balance during acute exacerbations are also related to changes in leptin metabolism as well as to the systemic inflammatory response (Creutzberg et al. 2000).

In summary, increases in REE and activity-related energy expenditure, as well as reduced dietary intake, can contribute to weight loss and muscle wasting in patients with COPD. Although the full spectrum of processes underlying the alterations in energy and substrate metabolism in COPD are incompletely understood, work of breathing, systemic inflammation, decreased mechanical efficiency of exercise and inefficient muscle metabolism likely all play a role, albeit potentially to different degrees and in different combinations in individual patients.

Nutritional intervention in COPD

Carbohydrate/fat

Most intervention strategies are directed to balance energy expenditure by administration of nutritional supplements. Meal-related dyspnoea and limited ventilatory reserves, however, may restrict the quantity and composition of nutritional support in patients with respiratory disease. Nutrient administration is associated with an obligate increase in ventilation and metabolic rate. The basis stoichiometry of fuel oxidation and storage indicates that the composition of the caloric intake can influence carbon dioxide production and therefore ventilatory demand. Oxidative combustion of glucose consumes 200 ml/min oxygen for each kcal of reactant, resulting in a net carbon dioxide production of 200 ml/min. The respiratory quotient (RQ or ratio carbon dioxide production/oxygen consumption) equals 1. The stoichiometric formula of fat oxidation is 0.71 indicating a lower-ventilatory load by reduced carbon dioxide production. Further evidence was derived from excessive carbon dioxide production by carbohydrate administration in mechanically ventilated patients (Talpers et al. 1992, Askanazi et al. 1980). However, these effects occur only in cases of excessive carbohydrate load, resulting in caloric overload. Under these circumstances, triglyceride biosynthesis can be expected. Several studies in clinically stable COPD patients have examined the effects of a carbohydrate load on functional capacity in the immediate postprandial period. Using a high-caloric, carbohydrate-rich supplement (920 kcal, 53 per cent carbohydrate) several studies reported significantly greater increases in minute ventilation, carbon dioxide elimination, oxygen consumption, RQ, arterial carbon dioxide tension and fatigue score, together with an increase in the distance walked, when compared to a fat-rich drink (Efthimiou et al. 1992, Frankfort et al. 1991). A drawback of these studies is the fact that the patients received a high-energy bolus, which made it impossible to investigate whether the metabolic and ventilatory effects resulted from the load or from the composition of the supplement. After a more physiological energy load (500 kcal) no difference in postprandial exercise capacity was shown between a high- versus a low-fat diet (Akrabawi et al. 1996). A meal with high fat content resulted in a significant delay in gastric emptying compared to feeding a meal with a moderate fat content (Akrabawi et al. 1996). There are clinical ramifications to delayed gastric emptying, especially in patients with COPD. Owing to the disease process itself, such patients already suffer from hyperinflation, a flattened diaphragm and a reduction in abdominal volume, which results in feelings of bloatedness, abdominal discomfort and early satiety. A significant delay in gastric emptying may lead to an extended time of abdominal distention, affecting diaphragmatic mobility and thoracic expansion. High-fat diets may also cause bloating, loose stools or diarrhoea and may thus create tolerance problems. It is of interest to note that in line with this point of view, in another study (Vermeeren et al. 2001) the change in dyspnoea post- versus preprandial was significantly less after a carbohydrate-rich nutritional supplement (250 kcal) compared to a comparable fat-rich supplement. Furthermore, meal-related oxyhemoglobin desaturation may limit caloric intake and contribute to meal-related dyspnoea in some patients, primarily in those that are hypoxemic at rest (Schols et al. 1991d). The degree of desaturation appears to depend on meal type, being significantly higher after a fat-rich warm meal compared to a carbohydrate-rich cold meal (Schols et al. 1991d).

Protein

The effects of wasting disease on protein metabolism are characterized by net protein catabolism owing to differences between protein synthesis and breakdown rates. This is seen in a negative nitrogen balance. The pathophysiological mechanisms of this catabolic reaction are related to disease severity. One study has shown in clinically stable patients with COPD that the negative nitrogen balance is associated mainly with a decreased protein synthesis rate, whereas protein breakdown is hardly affected (Morrison et al. 1988). In critical illness, however, net protein catabolic rate can be markedly stimulated by relatively higher increases in protein breakdown rates than in synthesis rates, resulting in a rapid decrease in FFM. It should be noted that the catabolic response is a net phenomenon. In some tissues (e.g. muscle) protein breakdown is clearly present, whereas in some organs (e.g. liver) mixed reactions may occur with increases in the synthesis rates of some proteins (e.g. acute-phase proteins) and decreases in the synthesis rates of others (e.g. albumin). Indeed, in clinically stable patients with COPD, decreased plasma concentrations of (non-essential) amino acids were correlated with an elevated REE and elevated values of the acute-phase protein LPS-binding protein (Pouw et al. 1998). The emphasis with respect to protein requirements in disease must be on optimal rather than minimal amounts of dietary proteins. Unfortunately, a clear clinical or physiological endpoint for the determination of optimal protein requirements is not available. Only studies documenting the effects of dietary protein content on nitrogen balance or on protein kinetics have been published in various conditions. The available data suggest that, in healthy subjects and in stable disease, protein synthesis is optimally stimulated during administration of 1.5g protein/kg/day. Similarly, although the catabolic effects of acute disease cannot be manipulated merely by nutrition, net protein catabolic rates in these conditions are lowered by administration of 1.5–2.0g protein/day (Hopkins et al. 1983). Administration of proteins exceeding this quantity results only in increased protein catabolism.

Outcome of nutritional intervention

Oral nutritional supplements

The first clinical trials to test the hypothesis that nutritional depletion contributes to a decline in function in patients with COPD included short-term in-patient nutritional intervention. In two studies (Wilson et al. 1986, Whittaker et al. 1990) a significant increase in body weight and respiratory muscle function was reported after two to three weeks of oral or enteral nutritional support. It was suggested that the effect of this short period of nutritional repletion may be related more to repletion of muscle water and potassium than to the constitution of muscle protein nitrogen. Besides, it is likely that an increase in cellular energy levels contributes more to an improved muscle strength over the short term than to an increase in nitrogen retention (Russell et al. 1983). Only one study addresses the immune response to short-term nutritional intervention in nine patients with advanced COPD (Fuenzalida et al. 1990). Refeeding and weight gain were associated with a significant increase in absolute lymphocyte count and with an increase in reactivity to skin test antigens after 21 days of refeeding.

Since then, several studies have investigated the effectiveness of nutritional therapy over a more prolonged intervention period, ranging from one to three months. One in-patient study (Rogers et al. 1992) and one outpatient study (Efthimiou et al. 1988) show significant improvement in respiratory and peripheral skeletal muscle function, exercise capacity and health-related quality of life after three months' oral supplementation by about 1,000 kcal daily. In three other outpatients studies, however, despite a similar nutritional supplementation regimen, the average weight gain was less than 1.5 kg in eight weeks (Otte et al. 1989, Knowles et al. 1988, Lewis et al. 1987). Besides non-compliance, the poor treatment response may be attributed, at least in part, to an inadequate assessment of energy requirements and to the observation that the patients were taking supplements instead of their regular meals.

Despite the positive outcome of nutritional repletion in a controlled setting, the progressive character of weight loss in COPD demands appropriate feeding strategies to allow sustained outpatient nutritional intervention. In order to be able to provide a sufficient energy supply, the effect of an aggressive nutritional support regimen was studied in patients with severe COPD and weight loss not responding to oral supplementation (Donahoe et al. 1994). Over a prolonged interval of four months, nocturnal enteral nutritional support via a percutaneous endoscopic gastrostomy tube was provided. The treated group had nightly enteral feeding adjusted to maintain a total daily caloric intake greater than two times measured resting metabolic rate for sustained weight gain. Despite the magnitude of the intervention, a mean weight gain of only 3.3 per cent (0.2 kg/week) was seen in the treated group. Weight gain appeared limited by the magnitude of the required caloric intake and by significant shifting of caloric intake between oral and enteral intake. Most of the increase in body weight was fat mass, and no significant improvement of physiological function was observed. The limited therapeutic impact of isolated aggressive nutritional support could be related to the absence of a comprehensive rehabilitative strategy or to the fact that the selected patients were not only in a hypermetabolic state but also hypercatabolic.

Nutrition and exercise

From a functional point of view it is obvious to combine nutritional support with exercise if possible. In another study (Schols et al. 1995) the effects of a daily nutritional supplement as an integrated part of a pulmonary rehabilitation programme resulted in significant weight gain (0.4 kg/week), despite a daily supplementation which was much less than in most previous outpatient studies. The combined treatment of nutritional support and exercise not only increased body weight but also resulted in a significant improvement of FFM and respiratory muscle strength. The clinical relevance of treatment response was shown in a post hoc survival analysis of this study, demonstrating that weight gain and increase in respiratory muscle strength were associated with significantly increased survival rates (Schols et al. 1998). Weight gain remained a significant predictor of mortality independent of baseline lung function and other risk factors, including age, gender, smoking and resting arterial blood gases. In view of the ventilatory limitation and the experienced symptoms, exercise in most rehabilitation settings consists of general physical training, with an emphasis on endurance exercise. Nutritional depletion, however, specifically impairs muscle strength. Studies in elderly subjects without pulmonary disease have shown that, in particular, strength training with nutritional support is superior to nutritional support alone in reaching an increase in fat-free mass. No data are yet available regarding the effects of nutritional support and strength training in depleted patients with chronic respiratory disease.

Timing of nutritional support

Most studies have investigated the effects of nutritional supplementation in clinically stable patients. Anamnestic data, however, indicate that in some patients weight loss follows a stepwise pattern, associated with acute (infectious) exacerbations. During an acute exacerbation, energy balance is often negative due to a further increase in REE, but particularly due to a temporarily dramatic decrease in dietary intake (Vermeeren et al. 1997). Furthermore, these patients may have an increased risk for protein breakdown that may limit the effectiveness of nutritional supplementation (Saudny-Unterberger et al. 1997). Factors contributing to weight loss and muscle wasting during an acute exacerbation include an increase in symptoms, more pronounced systemic inflammation, alterations in leptin metabolism, and the use of high doses of glucocorticoids. Saundy-Unterberger et al. show a positive effect of nutritional support during hospitalization for an acute exacerbation, but clearly more research is needed to evaluate the relative effectiveness of nutritional support during or immediately after an acute exacerbation (Saudny-Unterberger et al. 1997).

Practical implementation of nutritional support

Based on the current insights in the relationship between nutritional depletion and outcome in COPD, a flow chart for nutritional screening and therapy is presented here (Figure 10.1).

Simple screening can be performed based on repeated measurements of body weight. Patients are characterized by BMI and the presence or absence of involuntary weight loss. Nutritional supplementation is indicated for underweight patients (BMI <21 kg/m²). Involuntary weight loss in patients with a BMI <25 kg/m² should be treated to prevent further deterioration; involuntary weight loss in patients with a BMI>25 kg/m² should be monitored to assess whether it is progressive. If possible, measurement of fat free mass as an indirect measure of muscle mass may provide a more detailed screening of patients, since this allows identification of normal-weight patients with a depleted fat free mass who, even despite a normal body weight, should be considered for diet therapy.

Depending on the underlying cause of energy imbalance (decreased dietary intake or increased nutritional requirements), initial nutritional therapy may involve adaptations of the dietary behaviour and food pattern followed by implementation of nutritional supplements. Nutritional support should be given as energy dense supplements well divided during the day to avoid loss of appetite and adverse metabolic and ventilatory effects resulting from a high-caloric load. When feasible, the patients

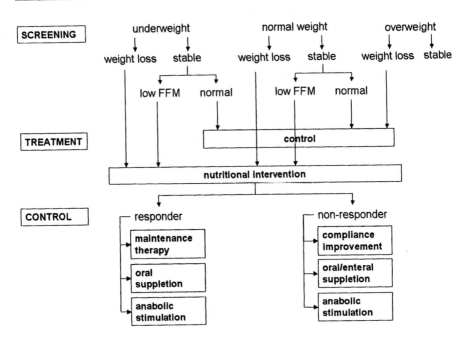

Figure 10.1 Flow chart for nutritional screening and therapy.

should be stimulated to follow an exercise programme. For the severely disabled cachectic patients unable to perform exercise training, even simple strength manoeuvres combined with ADL training and energy-conservation techniques may be effective. Exercise not only improves the effectiveness of nutritional therapy but also stimulates appetite. After four to eight weeks, therapy response can be determined. If weight gain and functional improvement are noted, the caregiver and the patient have to decide whether more improvement by a similar strategy is feasible or whether maintenance is the aim. It may then also be worthwhile to add to or alter the exercise training programme. If the desired response is not noted, it may be necessary to identify compliance issues. If compliance is not the problem, more calories may be needed by supplements or by enteral routes. Screening of nutritional status in relation to functional status can be done by the physician during hospitalization for an acute exacerbation during outpatient follow-up. The physician can consult the dietician for an insight into the cause and treatment of an impaired energy balance in weight-losing subjects and the physiotherapist for the type and intensity of an exercise programme. The respiratory nurse or nutritional therapist can play a valuable role in hospital and home care of patients with chronic lung disease during regular visits or phone calls. They can monitor compliance and the weight course during dietary therapy, give advice on meals and nutritional symptoms in the home setting to patients and their families, and feedback to the other caregivers. Despite an optimal implementation of nutritional therapy as part of an integrated treatment approach of COPD, one should recognize that even then a subgroup of patients may not achieve the intended effect due to the underlying mechanisms of weight loss that are yet unable to be reversed by mere caloric supplementation. Potential reversibility by means of specific nutrients (nutriceuticals) or pharmaceuticals will be a major focus of future research in this field.

Education

Human eating behaviour is shaped by many factors and is not easy to change, especially in the long term, which is necessary in the treatment of depletion in COPD patients. There are different factors, for example inadequate nutritional knowledge and misperceptions of eating pattern, that aggravate the essential changes to an improvement of dietary intake. Also, patients may experience negative reactions from their social environment to an increased intake of foods to elevate energy, since overeating is not regarded as socially desirable.

Nutritional education in Western countries has for decades been aimed at discouraging people from eating high-calorie foods and from frequent snacking, in order to contribute to prevention of cardiovascular disease, obesity and certain cancers. Frequently, eating high-calorie foods is therefore generally regarded as an unhealthy choice. Underweight COPD patients have to be persuaded to think and act differently. Behavioural strategies are necessary to provoke definitive changes in dietary patterns, and therefore a combination of dietary counselling and self-management is needed in patients with COPD. At this point, no data are available concerning education in changing eating habits in patients with COPD.

Conclusion

Chronic obstructive pulmonary disease is a major public health problem. Some of the targets of effective COPD management are to relieve symptoms and to improve health status as well as exercise intolerance and to reduce mortality. Nutritional supplementation therapy has to be considered as an effective treatment strategy in the integrated management of depleted or weight-losing patients with COPD.

References

Akrabawi SS, Mobarhan S, Stoltz RR et al. (1996) Gastric emptying, pulmonary function, gas exchange, and respiratory quotient after feeding a moderate versus high fat enteral formula meal in chronic obstructive pulmonary disease patients. Nutrition 12(4): 260–265.

Amoroso P, Wilson SR, Moxham J et al. (1993) Acute effects of inhaled salbutamol on the metabolic rate of normal subjects. Thorax 48(9): 882–885.

Anonymous (1983) Metropolitan Life Insurance Company. New weight standards for men and women. Bull Metropol Life Found 64: 1–4. Tables can be downloaded from http://www.halls.md/ideal-weight/met.htm.

Askanazi J, Elwyn DH, Silverberg PA et al. (1980) Respiratory distress secondary to a high carbohydrate load: a case report. Surgery 87(5): 596–598.

Baarends EM, Schols AM, van Marken Lichtenbelt WD et al. (1997a) Analysis of body water compartments in relation to tissue depletion in clinically stable patients with chronic obstructive pulmonary disease. American Journal of Clinical Nutrition 65(1): 88–94.

Baarends EM, Schols AM, Pannemans DL et al. (1997b) Total free living energy expenditure in patients with severe chronic obstructive pulmonary disease. American Journal of Respiratory and Critical Care Medicine 155(2): 549–54.

Baarends EM, Schols AM, Akkermans MA et al. (1997c) Decreased mechanical efficiency in clinically stable patients with COPD. Thorax 52(11): 981–986.

Baarends EM Schols AM, Nusmeier CM et al. (1998a) Breathing efficiency during inspiratory threshold loading in patients with chronic obstructive pulmonary disease. Clinical Physiology 18(3): 235–244.

Baarends EM, van Marken Lichtenbelt WD, Wouters EF et al. (1998b) Body-water compartments measured by bio-electrical impedance spectroscopy in patients with chronic obstructive pulmonary disease. Clinical Nutrition 17(1): 15–22.

Creutzberg EC, Schols AM, Bothmer-Quaedvlieg FC et al. (1998a) Prevalence of an elevated resting energy expenditure in patients with chronic obstructive pulmonary disease in relation to body composition and lung function. European Journal of Clinical Nutrition 52(6): 396–401.

Creutzberg EC, Schols AM, Bothmer-Quaedvlieg FC et al. (1998b) Acute effects of nebulized salbutamol on resting energy expenditure in patients with chronic obstructive pulmonary disease and in healthy subjects. Respiration 65(5): 375–380.

Creutzberg EC, Wouters EF, Vanderhoven-Augustin IM et al. (2000) Disturbances in leptin metabolism are related to energy imbalance during acute exacerbations of chronic obstructive pulmonary disease. American Journal of Respiratory and Critical Care Medicine 162(4 part 1): 1239–1245.

de Godoy I, Donahoe M, Calhoun WJ et al. (1996) Elevated TNF-alpha production by peripheral blood monocytes of weight-losing COPD patients. American Journal of Respiratory and Critical Care Medicine 153(2): 633–637.

Donahoe M, Mancino J, Costatino J et al. (1994) The effect of an aggressive support regimen on body composition in patients with severe COPD and weight loss. American Journal of Respiratory and Critical Care Medicine 149: A313.

Dornhurst AC (1955) Respiratory insufficiency. Lancet 11: 1185–1187.

Durnin JV, Womersley J (1974) Body fat assessed from total body density and its estimation from skinfold thickness: measurements on 481 men and women aged from 16 to 72 years. British Journal of Nutrition 32(1): 77–97.

Efthimiou J, Fleming J, Gomes C et al. (1988) The effect of supplementary oral nutrition in poorly nourished patients with chronic obstructive pulmonary disease. American Review of Respiratory Disease 137(5): 1075–1082.

Efthimiou J, Mounsey PJ, Benson DN et al. (1992) Effect of carbohydrate rich versus fat rich loads on gas exchange and walking performance in patients with chronic obstructive lung disease. Thorax 47(6): 451–456.

Engelen MP, Schols AM, Baken WC et al. (1994) Nutritional depletion in relation to respiratory and peripheral skeletal muscle function in outpatients with COPD. European Respiratory Journal 7(10): 1793–1797.

Engelen MP, Schols AM, Heidendal GA et al. (1998) Dual-energy X-ray absorptiometry in the clinical evaluation of body composition and bone mineral density in patients with chronic obstructive pulmonary disease. American Journal of Clinical Nutrition 68(6): 1298–1303.

Engelen MP, Schols AM, Does JD et al. (2000) Skeletal muscle weakness is associated with wasting of extremity fat-free mass but not with airflow obstruction in patients with chronic obstructive pulmonary disease. American Journal of Clinical Nutrition 71(3): 733–738.

Filley GF, Beckwitt HJ, Reeves JT et al. (1968) Chronic obstructive bronchopulmonary disease. American Journal of Medicine 44(1): 26–39.

Fowler J, Godlee R (1898) Emphysema of the Lungs. London: Longmans Green and Co.

Francia MD, Barbier D, Mege JL et al. (1994) Tumor necrosis factor-alpha levels and weight loss in chronic obstructive pulmonary disease. American Journal of Respiratory and Critical Care Medicine 150(5 Part 1): 1453–1455.

Frankfort JD, Fischer CE, Stansbury DW et al. (1991) Effects of high- and low-carbohydrate meals on maximum exercise performance in chronic airflow obstruction. Chest 100(3): 792–795.

Fuenzalida CE, Petty TL, Jones ML et al. (1990) The immune response to short-term nutritional intervention in advanced chronic obstructive pulmonary disease. American Review of Respiratory Disease 142(1): 49–56.

Goris AH, Vermeeren MA, Wouters EF et al. (2003) Energy balance in depleted ambulatory patients with chronic obstructive pulmonary disease: the effect of physical activity and oral nutritional supplementation. British Journal of Nutrition 89(5): 725–731.

Grunfeld C, Zhao C, Fuller J et al. (1996) Endotoxin and cytokines induce expression of leptin, the ob gene product, in hamsters. Journal of Clinical Investigation 97(9): 2152–2157.

Haarbo J, Gotfredsen A, Hassager C et al. (1991) Validation of body composition by dual energy X-ray absorptiometry (DEXA). Clinical Physiology 11(4): 331–341.

Harik-Khan RI, Fleg JL, Wise RA (2002) Body mass index and the risk of COPD. Chest 121(2): 370–376.

Hopkins B, Bristian B, Blackburn G (1983) Protein-Calorie Management in the Hospitalized Patient: Philadelphia, Pa: Harper & Row.

Hugli OS (1996) The daily energy expenditure in stable chronic obstructive pulmonary disease. American Journal of Respiratory and Critical Care Medicine 153(1): 294–300.

Hugli O, Schutz Y, Fitting JW (1995) The cost of breathing in stable chronic obstructive pulmonary disease. Clinical Science 89(6): 625–632.

Hunter AM, Carey MA, Larsh HW (1981) The nutritional status of patients with chronic obstructive pulmonary disease. American Review of Respiratory Disease 124(4): 376–381.

Jensen MD, Kanaley JA, Roust LR et al. (1993) Assessment of body composition with use of dual-energy x-ray absorptiometry: evaluation and comparison with other methods. Mayo Clinic Proceedings 68(9): 867–873.

Jounieaux V, Mayeux I (1995) Oxygen cost of breathing in patients with emphysema or chronic bronchitis in acute respiratory failure. American Journal of Respiratory and Critical Care Medicine 152(6 Part 1): 2181–2184.

Knowles JB, Fairbarn MS, Wiggs BJ et al. (1988) Dietary supplementation and respiratory muscle performance in patients with COPD. Chest 93(5): 977–983.

Landbo C, Prescott E, Lange P et al. (1999) Prognostic value of nutritional status in chronic obstructive pulmonary disease. American Journal of Respiratory and Critical Care Medicine 160(6): 1856–1861.

Lewis MI, Belman MJ, Dorr Uyemura L (1987) Nutritional supplementation in ambulatory patients with chronic obstructive pulmonary disease. American Review of Respiratory Disease 135(5): 1062–1068.

Lukaski HC (1987) Methods for the assessment of human body composition: traditional and new. American Journal of Clinical Nutrition 46(4): 537–556.

Lukaski HC, Johnson PE, Bolonchuk WW et al. (1985) Assessment of fat-free mass using bioelectrical impedance measurements of the human body. American Journal of Clinical Nutrition 41(4): 810–817.

Mannix ET, Manfredi F, Palange P et al. (1992) The effect of oxygen with exercise on atrial natriuretic peptide in chronic obstructive lung disease. Chest 10(2): 341–344.

Mazess RB, Barden HS, Bisek JP et al. (1990) Dual-energy x-ray absorptiometry for total-body and regional bone-mineral and soft-tissue composition. American Journal of Clinical Nutrition 51(6): 1106–1112.

Morrison WL, Gibson JN, Scrimgeour C et al. (1988) Muscle wasting in emphysema. Clinical Science 75(4): 415–420.

Nguyen LT, Bedu M, Caillaud D et al. (1999) Increased resting energy expenditure is related to plasma TNF-alpha concentration in stable COPD patients. Clinical Nutrition 18(5): 269–274.

Otte KE, Ahlburg P, Stellfeld M (1989) Nutritional repletion in malnourished patients with emphysema. Journal of Parenteral and Enteral Nutrition 13(2): 152–156.

Pouw EM, Schols AM, Deutz NE et al. (1998) Plasma and muscle amino acid levels in relation to resting energy expenditure and inflammation in stable chronic obstructive pulmonary disease. American Journal of Respiratory and Critical Care Medicine 158(3): 797–801.

Rogers RM, Donahoe M, Costantino J (1992) Physiologic effects of oral supplemental feeding in malnourished patients with chronic obstructive pulmonary disease: a randomized control study. American Review of Respiratory Disease 146(6): 1511–1517.

Russell DM, Prendergast PJ, Darby PL et al. (1983) A comparison between muscle function and body composition in anorexia nervosa: the effect of refeeding. American Journal of Clinical Nutrition 38(2): 229–237.

Saudny-Unterberger H, Martin JG, Gray-Donald K (1997) Impact of nutritional support on functional status during an acute exacerbation of chronic obstructive pulmonary disease. American Journal of Respiratory and Critical Care Medicine 156(3 Part 1): 794–799.

Schols AM (1999) TNF-alpha and hypermetabolism in chronic obstructive pulmonary disease. Nutrition 18(5): 255–257.

Schols AM, Dingemans AM, Soeters PB et al. (1990) Within-day variation of bioelectrical resistance measurements in patients with chronic obstructive pulmonary disease. Clinical Nutrition 9: 266–271.

Schols AM, Wouters EF, Soeters PB et al. (1991a) Body composition by bioelectrical-impedance analysis compared with deuterium dilution and skinfold anthropometry in patients with chronic obstructive pulmonary disease. American Journal of Clinical Nutrition 53(2): 421–424.

Schols AM, Fredrix EW, Soeters PB et al. (1991b) Resting energy expenditure in patients with chronic obstructive pulmonary disease. American Journal of Clinical Nutrition 54(6): 983–987.

Schols AM, Mostert R, Soeters PB et al. (1991c) Energy balance in patients with chronic obstructive pulmonary disease. American Review of Respiratory Disease 143(6): 1248–1252.

Schols AM Mostert R, Cobben N et al. (1991d) Transcutaneous oxygen saturation and carbon dioxide tension during meals in patients with chronic obstructive pulmonary disease. Chest 100(5): 1287–1292.

Schols AM, Soeters PB, Dingemans AM et al. (1993) Prevalence and characteristics of nutritional depletion in patients with stable COPD eligible for pulmonary rehabilitation. American Review of Respiratory Disease 147(5): 1151–1156.

Schols AM, Soeters PB, Mostert R et al. (1995) Physiologic effects of nutritional support and anabolic steroids in patients with chronic obstructive pulmonary disease. A placebo-controlled randomized trial. American Journal of Respiratory and Critical Care Medicine 152(4 Part 1): 1268–1274.

Schols AM, Buurman WA, Staal van den Brekel AJ et al. (1996) Evidence for a relation between metabolic derangements and increased levels of inflammatory mediators in a subgroup of patients with chronic obstructive pulmonary disease. Thorax 51(8): 819–824.

Schols AM, Slangen J, Volovics L et al. (1998) Weight loss is a reversible factor in the prognosis of chronic obstructive pulmonary disease. American Journal of Respiratory and Critical Care Medicine 157(6 Part 1): 1791–1797.

Schols AM, Creutzberg EC, Buurman WA et al. (1999) Plasma leptin concentration is related to pro-inflammatory status and dietary intake in patients with COPD. American Journal of Respiratory and Critical Care Medicine 160(4): 1220–1226.

Soeters PB, Von Meyenfeldt MF, Meijerink WJ et al. (1990) Serum albumin and mortality. Lancet 335(8685): 348–351.

Sridhar MK, Carter R, Lean ME et al. (1994) Resting energy expenditure and nutritional state of patients with increased oxygen cost of breathing due to emphysema, scoliosis and thoracoplasty. Thorax 49(8): 781–785.

Takabatake N, Nakamura H, Abe S et al. (1999) Circulating leptin in patients with chronic obstructive pulmonary disease. American Journal of Respiratory and Critical Care Medicine 159(4 Part 1): 1215–1219.

Talpers SS, Romberger DJ, Bunce SB et al. (1992) Nutritionally associated increased carbon dioxide production. Excess total calories vs. high proportion of carbohydrate calories. Chest 102(2): 551–555.

Tuten MB, Wogt S, Dasse F et al. (1985) Utilization of prealbumin as a nutritional parameter. Journal of Parenteral and Enteral Nutrition 9(6): 709–711.

Vandenbergh E, Woestijne van de KP, Gyselen A (1967) Weight changes in the terminal stages of chronic obstructive pulmonary disease. American Review of Respiratory Disease 95(4): 556–566.

Vermeeren MA, Schols AM, Wouters EF (1997) Effects of an acute exacerbation on nutritional and metabolic profile of patients with COPD. European Respiratory Journal 10(10): 2264–2269.

Vermeeren MA, Wouters EF, Nelissen LH et al. (2001) Acute effects of different nutritional supplements on symptoms and functional capacity in patients with chronic obstructive pulmonary disease. American Journal of Clinical Nutrition 73(2): 295–301.

Whittaker JS, Ryan CF, Buckley PA et al. (1990) The effects of refeeding on peripheral and respiratory muscle function in malnourished chronic obstructive pulmonary disease patients. American Review of Respiratory Disease 142(2): 283–288.

Wilson DO, Rogers RM, Sanders MH et al. (1986) Nutritional intervention in malnourished patients with emphysema. American Review of Respiratory Disease 134(4): 672–677.

Wilson DO, Rogers RM, Wright EC et al. (1989) Body weight in chronic obstructive pulmonary disease. The National Institutes of Health Intermittent Positive-Pressure Breathing Trial. American Review of Respiratory Disease 139(6): 1435–1438.

Wilson SR, Amoroso P, Moxham J et al. (1993) Modification of the thermogenic effect of acutely inhaled salbutamol by chronic inhalation in normal subjects. Thorax 48(9): 886–889.

Wuyam B, Payen JF, Levy P et al. (1992) Metabolism and aerobic capacity of skeletal muscle in chronic respiratory failure related to chronic obstructive pulmonary disease. European Respiratory Journal 5(2): 157–162.

Chapter 11
Cost-effectiveness of pulmonary rehabilitation

T. GRIFFITHS

Introduction

As the clinical effectiveness of pulmonary rehabilitation is now well established, the imperative has been to translate the results obtained in the subjects of randomized controlled trials into health gains for people with chronic respiratory disability generally. In establishing new services, we cannot avoid issues of resource allocation. With a limited budget, how can resources be directed to those interventions that are both effective and good value for money? Those who commission health care will wish to have an indication of the likely expenditure involved for any intervention, together with the benefits to patients and the health service that might be obtained. It is these issues of cost and benefit that are addressed by studies which include estimates of the cost of providing the service together with clinical and health resource usage outcomes. The overall cost of including a particular intervention in the care of patients with any disease will incorporate both the cost of providing the service and the subsequent effect on the cost of caring for the patient in terms of drugs used, primary- and secondary-care consultations, hospital admissions experienced, etc. However, the majority of studies of pulmonary rehabilitation published to date have reported only partial costings of providing the service, and many have not measured the cost of subsequent changes in health care usage. A number of studies have used surrogate measures of subsequent cost/benefit, such as hospital admission rates.

The major component of the cost of providing health services to patients with chronic obstructive pulmonary disease (COPD) is the cost of acute medical emergency admissions (Calverley and Belamy 2000). Hence, many studies have concentrated on hospital admission rates in the post-rehabilitation period as a primary outcome – frequently compared with the pre-rehabilitation period. A problem with this approach is that rehabilitation may affect not only admission rates but also length of stay. Additionally, while investigators may provide a point estimate of the number of admissions or hospital days avoided, and the cost of the

173

programme, very few have given an indication of the precision of these estimates or performed any kind of sensitivity analysis on the cost effects of the intervention. More recently, randomized controlled trials have been published that have simultaneously investigated the incremental cost and effect of adding multidisciplinary pulmonary rehabilitation to standard care and performed sensitivity analyses with indications of the precision of estimates of cost-effectiveness.

This chapter will review key studies of rehabilitation in in-patient, out-patient and community settings that provide information on:

- **direct cost**: the cost to the health service of providing a rehabilitation programme
- **cost/benefit**: effects of rehabilitation on the overall cost of caring for patients with COPD
- **cost-effectiveness**: the cost of rehabilitation in relation to the clinical benefits obtained
- **cost/utility**: the cost of rehabilitation in relation to the quantity and patient-centred value that rehabilitation can add to the lives of patients.

Direct cost

A major problem in the interpretation of the cost of providing a rehabilitation programme is that the programmes described in the literature have a differing content and are undertaken in different countries and health care systems. However, a number of authors have reported the cost of providing their rehabilitation programme. The point estimates of cost per patient rehabilitated and cost per session of rehabilitation are given in Table 11.1. In this table, no attempt has been made to allow for changes in inflation and differential exchange rates over time.

The first full-cost analysis of pulmonary rehabilitation came from a programme in Loma Linda, California (Burton et al. 1975) and involved 80 patients undergoing an individually tailored multidisciplinary pulmonary rehabilitation programme with both in-patient and outpatient elements. The estimated expenditure on the programme for the 80 patients was fully costed and found to be $36,160 a year – an average of $452 per patient a year at 1982 values. Later, a study carried out in Seattle, Washington (Holle et al. 1988) showed improved exercise capacity following an outpatient-based programme incorporating home exercise, breathing training and respiratory muscle training. The authors reported that the cost of this six-week, one-session-a-week intervention was $600 to $800 per patient. A similar programme of ten weeks' duration was subsequently reported from Newark, New Jersey (Reina-Rosenbaum et al. 1997). Their intervention included one hospital-based session a week with multidisciplinary input, together with a programme of daily exercise and respiratory muscle training at home. Significant improvements were

Table 11.1 Comparison of reported direct cost per patient of providing pulmonary rehabilitation programmes

Study reference	Country	Setting	Duration (weeks)	Number of observed sessions	Cost	Cost per observed session
Burton et al. 1975	USA	outpatient**	Variable	Variable	$452	N/A
Holle et al. 1988	USA	outpatient*	6	6	$600–$800	$100–$133
Goldstein et al. 1997	USA	in-patient and outpatient**	24 total	N/A	CA$10,228	N/A
Wijkstra et al. 2000	Netherlands	community	72	84	$2300	$27
Reina-Rosenbaum et al. 1997	USA	outpatient**	10	10	$650	$65
White et al. 1997	UK	outpatient**	6	12	£400	£33
Singh et al. 1998	UK	outpatient**	7	14	£422	£30
Griffiths et al. 2001	UK	outpatient**	6	18	£725	£40
Troosters et al. 2000	Belgium	outpatient*	24	72	$2615	$36

The cost figures are those reported by the authors at the time of their publication.
*Primarily muscle training programme **Multidisciplinary programme N/A not appropriate

observed at the end of the programme in exercise performance and dyspnoea. The estimated cost of this programme was $650.

Two reports from different centres in the UK estimated the cost per patient of providing outpatient rehabilitation to be £422 for a seven-week, 14-session multidisciplinary programme in Leicester (Singh et al. 1998) and £400 for a six-week, 12-session, multidisciplinary programme in Bristol (White et al. 1997). Both of these costings were set alongside significant beneficial changes in walking ability and disease-specific health status. Subsequently, a prospective randomized controlled trial of a six-month, three-session-a-week outpatient programme of endurance and strength training in patients with COPD was reported from Belgium (Troosters et al. 2000). The exercise programme was effective in improving exercise tolerance and quality of life as compared with a control group. The direct cost of providing the programme was estimated from reimbursed charges by the Belgian National Health Insurance. This amounted to $2615 (standard deviation $625) per programme per patient.

From a randomized controlled trial of a six-week, three-session-per-week multidisciplinary rehabilitation programme reported by Griffiths et al. (Griffiths et al. 2000), the accompanying health economics data were reported one year later (Griffiths 2001). The programme included elements of exercise reconditioning, education, dietetic support, stress management and relaxation training. The programme was delivered by dedicated occupational therapy, physiotherapy, dietetic, medical and clerical staff. The cost of the programme was determined from staff costs, equipment and consumables, travel and institutional overheads. The programme had the capacity to rehabilitate 20 patients in each six-week period, but the costs were estimated conservatively as if the programme actually ran with 17 patients to reflect the fact that all programmes see patients dropping out of rehabilitation. The estimated cost of providing this programme, which showed important functional and health-status benefits, was £725 per patient. The contribution of the various components to this cost is shown in Figure 11.1. In this, as in other outpatient studies, the staff costs form the main component of the overall direct expenditure involved in providing pulmonary rehabilitation.

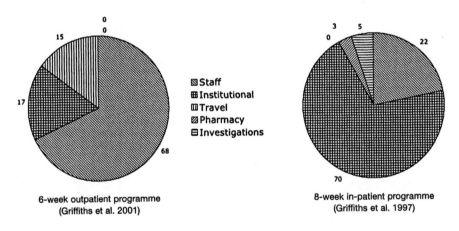

6-week outpatient programme
(Griffiths et al. 2001)

8-week in-patient programme
(Griffiths et al. 1997)

Figure 11.1 Cost components in providing pulmonary rehabilitation in outpatient and in-patient programmes.

At the opposite end of the spectrum of rehabilitation cost are programmes with an in-patient component. The programme of this type that has been most thoroughly costed was from Canada (Goldstein et al. 1994, Goldstein et al. 1997). The programme consisted of an initial eight-week, in-patient phase (Monday to Friday) followed by four months of gradually reducing outpatient support. The in-patient phase included exercise training, patient education and psychosocial support, recreational activities and relaxation classes. The outpatient phase consisted of a home exercise regimen and gradually reducing frequency of contact with the centre. Home visits by rehabilitation staff were also a part of this phase.

Patients undergoing this programme displayed significantly better improvements in functional and health status than those in the control group. The costing of the programme was highly detailed and included hotel costs, investigation costs, medications, institutional support and overheads, staff and transport. The direct cost of providing the in-patient phase of rehabilitation amounted to Canadian $10,228 per patient. The proportionate contributions of the various components of the cost are shown in Figure 11.1 above. It is clear that the largest contribution to the cost of in-patient rehabilitation relates to hotel services provided by the hospital. For this reason, in-patient rehabilitation is the most expensive mode of rehabilitation to deliver. However, it has been argued (unpublished communications) that for some patients this may be the modality most likely to produce improvement.

The community setting for pulmonary rehabilitation has also been considered economically. A study (Wijkstra et al. 1995, Wijkstra et al. 1996) from the Netherlands reported the outcomes of a prolonged community-based rehabilitation programme. Patients visited a local physiotherapist once a week or once a month for 18 months after a three-month, two-a-week, community-based programme. Although numbers in this study were small, a once-a-month continuation programme appeared to be the more effective strategy when compared to controls, but not statistically different from a once-a-week follow-up strategy. Retrospectively the authors estimated the cost of weekly community-based follow-up and compared that to an estimate of what costs might have been for a similarly intense programme if individual patients had received follow-up in hospital. The resulting estimates, given in a later review article (Wijkstra et al. 2000), were that the overall direct cost of providing 18 months' community-based rehabilitation with a locally available physiotherapy facility was $2,300, while outpatient-based care might have cost $4,250 per patient. They stated that the difference in cost largely represented travel involved in attending the hospital. However, it should be noted that had the follow-up in hospital occurred in a group setting as is the usual practice, the projected cost of outpatient follow-up might have been considerably lower. The sensitivity of economic analysis to differences such as this emphasizes the need for future randomized trials to address issues of differences in cost and outcome of rehabilitation in different settings.

As yet no prospective cost analysis comparing in-patient, outpatient and community-based rehabilitation has been reported. Indeed, differences in national health services make the results of health economic studies of pulmonary rehabilitation difficult to generalize.

Cost/benefit

Cost/benefit analysis is used to assess the overall effect on cost to the health service of adding a given intervention to patients' care. In order to carry this out fully, the cost of the intervention should be known together with an assessment of the downstream effects on the cost of patient care. Many studies have reported the effect of rehabilitation on health service usage, e.g. post-rehabilitation hospital admissions, but few have costed both the intervention and the cost of subsequent care.

Reduction in the use of hospital care by rehabilitation graduates was one of the earliest benefits of pulmonary rehabilitation to be reported, and was recognized as indicating that rehabilitation might indeed be cost-beneficial, i.e. reduce the cost of caring for patients. The first major study to report health service usage as an outcome came from Denver, Colorado (Petty et al. 1969). In this study, 182 patients with emphysema or chronic bronchitis with an average FEV_1 of 0.94L entered a programme of outpatient rehabilitation which included graded exercise allied to comprehensive in-patient care for those who suffered an exacerbation during the intervention period. The experience of hospital admission was compared between the year prior to entering the programme and in the first year thereafter. A substantial (48 per cent) reduction was seen in days spent in hospital, with eight people returned to work after more than a year of unemployment. These results, though impressive and triggering further research, did not give a reliable estimate of the contribution of outpatient-based rehabilitation to the reduction in hospitalization as there was no control group. This ground-breaking report was followed by a report on the ongoing hospital admission requirements for respiratory disease of their patients (Hudson et al. 1976). The number of days patients spent in hospital in each of the four years after entering this comprehensive outpatient programme was compared with their experience in the year leading up to entering the programme. The first 113 patients entering their multimodality programme were given a questionnaire in which to record their recollection of hospital admissions. The results of this study suggest that considerable reductions in hospital usage were seen in patients following rehabilitation. While the study does not include a comparison non-rehabilitated group, the effect was thought likely to be of economic importance.

The study from Loma Linda (Burton et al. 1975) followed 80 patients undergoing a rehabilitation programme with both in-patient and outpatient elements for five years. Their experience of hospital admission following admission to the programme was compared retrospectively with their admission record in the preceding one-year period. In the year before rehabilitation, the cohort spent 17.41 days in hospital and in the years after entering rehabilitation, 7.78, 4.91, 2.74, 2.22 and 3.26 in each of the five succeeding years. The cost of a hospital bed per day was assigned a value of $400, and the estimated cost of rehabilitation was $452 per patient. From these figures, notional savings in cost were estimated for their programme with a reduction of cost of $308,160 in the first year. Unfortunately, no indication of the statistical precision of these estimates was given in this report, the findings were not subjected to statistical analysis, and there was no non-rehabilitation comparison group. Despite the lack of a control group, it does seem likely that this study indicated a reduction in health service usage following entry into ongoing pulmonary rehabilitation.

In an observational study of 61 patients with chronic disability from COPD or asthma reported from Italy (Foglio et al. 1999), the effect of out-patient rehabilitation on hospital usage was reported. The subjects underwent three outpatient sessions a week for eight to ten weeks. The programme included upper- and lower-limb training, disease-specific education, and nutritional and psychological support as indicated. Follow-up was for 12 months. Significant improvements occurred from baseline to follow-up in exercise tolerance and health status. Hospital admissions were compared for the two years prior to entering rehabilitation and for the year after intervention. In asthmatics, the average annual admission rate fell significantly from 0.9 (SD 0.7) admissions a year for the year before rehabilitation to 0.03 (0.2) in the year after. For COPD patients the change was from 0.8 (0.7) to 0.1 (0.3) admissions a year, p (probability) = 0.005. While this was not a controlled trial, the authors showed that the admission rate for their subjects was stable in the two years before rehabilitation without an excess of admissions in the year immediately before rehabilitation. The suggestion was, therefore, that rehabilitation could reduce secondary-care usage in the period after an effective programme.

Although not characterized as community-based pulmonary rehabilitation, reports of comprehensive home-care programmes for patients with COPD have been described in the literature. In a retrospective study from Pittsburgh, Pennsylvania (Roselle and D'Amico 1982), home respiratory therapy support (amounting effectively to a rehabilitation programme) for up to 12 months found that the average number of hospital admissions fell significantly from 1.28, with an average length of stay of 18.25 days in the year before entering the programme, to 0.48 with an average length of stay of 6.09 days in the first year after entry. This led the authors to estimate a reduction in cost of $2,625 per patient a year in this programme. Retrospective analysis of another home care programme in Norwalk, Connecticut (Haggerty et al. 1991), which analysed symmetrical time periods before and after entry to the programme, also suggests cost savings as a result of reduction in secondary-care usage in the time after entry compared with the period before intervention. The estimated cost reduction was $328 per patient per month.

A major criticism of all the studies so far described is that patients may have been more likely to enter the programme as a result of a period of ill health and therefore be liable to record lesser periods of hospitalization following recovery. Additionally, the statistical problem of regression to the mean makes retrospective studies of pre- to post-rehabilitation changes, with no control groups, impossible to interpret in terms of quantifying their true effect on health service usage or health service costs. A major randomized controlled trial that addressed these issues was carried out in San Diego, California (Ries et al. 1995), in which 119 subjects were randomized to a 12-session, eight-week, multidisciplinary pro-gramme of rehabilitation, followed by monthly reinforcement sessions for a year, or to a purely educational programme. Participants were followed for four years. Although there was a trend towards a reduction in days spent in hospital in the multidisciplinary rehabilitation group, there was no statistically significant difference found when compared with changes in the control group. The authors suggest that this difference compared with earlier studies may have, in part, arisen from changes that had occurred in hospitalization patterns for COPD with time. However, it is also true that the inclusion of a control group would have excluded the effect of regression to the mean on recorded outcomes. Further studies were needed to elucidate whether pulmonary rehabilitation reduced health care usage and costs.

Two randomized controlled trials have directly investigated the effect on cost of adding pulmonary rehabilitation to standard care (Goldstein et al. 1997, Griffiths et al. 2001). The study from Goldstein et al. provided data on the cost/benefits of in-patient rehabilitation (Goldstein et al. 1997). This was done by analysing the cost of care for patients over six months in their rehabilitation and standard care groups (Goldstein et al. 1994). They showed greater costs associated with two months of in-patient rehabilitation followed by four months of home support than in the standard care group. The only areas where costs were less in the reha-bilitated group were prescribed drugs and community services. Overall, the average cost of adding their rehabilitation programme to standard care (incremental cost) was Canadian $11,597 per patient. The authors did not report any data on hospital admissions unrelated to rehabilitation itself that may have occurred during the study period. Additionally, patients were excluded if they suffered a prolonged exacerbation. Thus, it is not possible to gauge whether this programme might have affected hos-pitalization or increased resource utilization associated with any subsequent exacerbations.

The issue of downstream health service usage was subsequently addressed in the study of Griffiths et al. (2001). In this study, the cost of providing rehabilitation and also the cost of overall patient care was esti-mated for the year after entering rehabilitation. This study took the form of a randomized controlled trial and so the incremental cost of adding rehabilitation could be determined. Their 18-session, multidisciplinary, outpatient rehabilitation programme did not alter the number of patients requiring at least one admission in the year after entering the programme. However, in those patients needing hospital in-patient care, the total number of hospital admissions was reduced and the average number of days spent in hospital was halved. The saving in hospital bed-days was equivalent to a saving of about four bed-days per patient rehabilitated. Benefits were also seen in primary-care usage with a significant reduction in home visits and an increase in surgery visits in the rehabilitated group. The authors speculate that rehabilitation might have led to fitness and behaviour changes enabling patients to seek timely help at the GP's surgery when they needed attention. With notional costs for a hospital bed-day of £195, GP home visit of £30 and a GP surgery consultation of £10 and with no significant differences in drug costs between the control and rehabilitation groups, the average, overall cost of caring for patients for a year with and without rehabilitation was calculated. It was estimated that standard care cost £1,826 a year, and care including rehabilitation cost £1,674. The £150 difference between the two strategies was not statistically significant. These findings suggest that overall, including outpatient rehabilitation, the care of chronically disabled patients is likely to be cost neutral to the health service, the cost of rehabilitation being recouped by downstream reductions in health service usage.

From the evidence available, we can conclude that pulmonary rehabilitation results in a reduction in later health service resource utilization. In-patient programmes are unlikely to be cost-beneficial, because of the major contribution to costs of the in-patient stay. Outpatient programmes, on the other hand, provide a cost-neutral way to enhance the health of patients with chronic respiratory disability. More work is needed to compare the cost/benefits of rehabilitation in different environments – particularly in hospital and community settings.

Cost-effectiveness

Whereas cost/benefit analysis balances the cost of adding the intervention with any cost reductions that might ensue, cost-effectiveness analysis balances the cost of the intervention against clinical outcomes and estimates the cost of obtaining a given degree of clinical benefit to patients. To carry out this kind of analysis, a detailed incremental cost of adding the intervention to standard care must be determined, together with robust incremental outcome measurement.

A useful measure of programme effectiveness that has been reported in the two major health economic analyses of pulmonary rehabilitation (Goldstein et al. 1997, Griffiths et al. 2001) is the number needed to treat (NNT). Using this outcome, it is recognized that not all patients in the rehabilitation group will achieve a clinically important benefit and that some of the patients in the control group may show benefit with time alone. To use this outcome, a parallel group, randomized, controlled trial study design is needed. The inverse of the difference in the proportion of patients achieving a clinically important benefit in the control and rehabilitation groups is the NNT. This is, in effect, the number of patients that would need to be offered rehabilitation to gain one more patient obtaining a clinically important benefit than would be found with standard care alone.

The more effective the programme, the greater the proportion of graduates that will achieve clinically important benefit when compared with their control groups. If the average incremental cost of rehabilitation per patient is multiplied by the NNT, the product is the programme's cost to provide one patient with a minimal clinically important benefit – an index of cost-effectiveness. The studies used the same disease-specific health status measure (the chronic respiratory disease questionnaire) (Guyatt et al. 1987). This instrument has domains of dyspnoea, fatigue, emotion and mastery. A change in the average score for each item in these domains of 0.5 is accepted as indicating a clinically relevant change. Thus, for each domain, the NNT to achieve this level of benefit at the end of the intervention is determined. The findings of cost-effectiveness in the two existing studies using this method are shown in Table 11.2. Direct comparison between the two programmes is not possible, as the patient groups, health services, styles of rehabilitation, and timing of outcome measurement in relation to intensive rehabilitation are different. In order to quantify differences in cost-effectiveness between different programme formats, further randomized trials addressing the question are needed.

Table 11.2 Cost-effectiveness analysis using NNT for an in-patient and an outpatient rehabilitation programme

Health domain*	In-patient (Goldstein et al. 1997)		Outpatient (Griffiths et al. 2001)	
	NNT	Cost (£)	NNT	Cost (£)
Dyspnoea	4.1	19,407	2.3	1,730
Fatigue	4.4	20,822	2.5	1,880
Emotion	3.3	15,617	2.2	1,654
Mastery	2.5	11,830	2.9	2,181

*From the chronic respiratory disease questionnaire (Guyatt et al. 1987)

Cost/utility

Cost/utility analysis is a particular form of cost-effectiveness analysis. Here, the effectiveness outcome is a measure of the value placed by people on the benefits that may accrue from rehabilitation. This may be further refined by also taking into account the duration of life achieved following an intervention. As utility outcomes are generic rather than disease-specific, cost/utility analysis can be used to compare cost-effectiveness across different interventions and different diseases.

Indices of utility may be derived from generic health status questionnaires for which the health states defined by a subject's responses have been ranked in terms of preference by a reference population. In this way a notional value (or utility) placed on a subject's health state can be assigned from zero (least-valued health state) to one (most-valued health state). This process gives a measure of the 'quality' of life, and can be combined with a measure of the quantity of life, i.e. survival. The Quality Adjusted Life Year (QALY) is the mathematical product of the utility score and the duration of life for the individual. Thus, one year of life lived with a utility score of 0.75 would result in 0.75 QALYs being produced.

In a parallel group randomized controlled trial setting, the costs of care and the QALYs produced during follow-up can be determined for each individual. It is then possible to estimate the incremental cost of adding an intervention such as rehabilitation to standard care together with the incremental effect on utility expressed as QALYs. The mean number of QALYs generated by the intervention and control groups and the overall costs expended on the two groups can be used to produce an incremental cost/utility ratio according to the following equation:

$$R = \frac{\bar{C}_T - \bar{C}_C}{\bar{U}_T - \bar{U}_C} = \frac{\Delta\bar{C}}{\Delta\bar{U}}$$

where R is the incremental cost/utility ratio, $\bar{C}_C$ and $\bar{U}_C$ are the means of the control group costs (in pounds sterling) and utility (in QALYs) respectively, $\bar{C}_T$ and $\bar{U}_T$ are the means of the treatment group costs and utility respectively. $\Delta\bar{C}$ and $\Delta\bar{U}$ are the incremental cost and incremental utility respectively. The cost/utility ratio provides a point estimate of the mean overall cost for each QALY gained by adding rehabilitation to standard care.

In the randomized controlled trial of outpatient rehabilitation by Griffiths et al. (2000, 2001), this approach to cost/utility analysis was taken. The measure of health status used was the SF-6D (Brazier et al. 1998). This is a restructuring of some of the responses to the SF-36 questionnaire to give a health state for each individual subject. The health states represented by the SF-6D have a value (utility) from 0 (least-desirable health state) to 1 (most-desirable health state) as determined by a reference population. Follow-up was for one year, and the date of death of any participants in the study was recorded. Twelve of the 101 patients in the control group and six of the 99 patients in the rehabilitation group died during the year of follow-up (difference not statistically significant). From the duration of life and utility scores, the QALYs accrued by each subject were calculated. In the year of follow-up, QALYs gained in the standard care group were 0.351 (SD 0.08) and in the rehabilitated group 0.381 (SD 0.01). The difference between the groups was statistically significant (p = 0.03). The cost/utility ratio was calculated as above. As the point estimate of incremental cost was –£152 (95% CI – 880 to 577), the point estimate of the cost per QALY gained in this study was negative, i.e. valued life was gained by rehabilitation at no additional overall cost to the health service. Because the cost/utility ratio is not normally distributed, it is necessary to estimate the statistical precision of its value non-parametrically. The authors did this using the 'bootstrap' technique, which involves statistical modelling. They concluded that the probability that the true cost/utility ratio fell below £0 per QALY was 0.64. The probability that the true cost per QALY was less than £3000 was 0.74, and the probability the cost per QALY was below £10,000 was 0.9.

Where health budgets are finite, decision-makers have to decide how a limited pot of money will be spent. One of the factors that will affect this decision-making is the level of health gain that will accrue by investing in different forms of health care. Cost/utility ratios in terms of cost per QALY gained have been used to compare the effectiveness of investing sums of money in different treatments for different diseases. In this context, multidisciplinary, outpatient, pulmonary rehabilitation that is likely to have a negative cost per QALY ratio has been compared with other interventions, such as hip replacement surgery (£1,180 per QALY), coronary artery bypass graft (£2,090 per QALY), hospital haemodialysis (£21,970 per QALY) and treating hypertension with beta-blockade in middle-aged men and women (£26,796 and £67,678 per QALY respectively) (Griffiths et al. 2001). Such comparisons will inevitably have an effect on purchasing decisions in the health service.

Conclusion

The evidence base on which pulmonary rehabilitation stands is now extensive. Evidence of its health economic effects has always formed a strand in the available literature that has indicated health-economic benefits. This has culminated in the recent interest in rigorous health economic evaluation, in light of which we can begin to draw conclusions:

- The cost/benefits of rehabilitation will depend crucially on the setting of rehabilitation.
- In-patient programmes tend to increase overall cost of care.
- Pulmonary rehabilitation produces health benefits at costs generally regarded as good value for money and hence should be regarded as cost-effective.
- Outpatient programmes are probably cost-beneficial to the health service.
- The evidence fully justifies widespread investment in pulmonary rehabilitation services for patients disabled by chronic lung disease.

References

Brazier J, Usherwood T, Harper R et al. (1998) Deriving a preference-based single index from the UK SF-36 Health Survey. Journal of Clinical Epidemiology 51(11): 1115–1128.

Burton GG, Gee G, Hodgkin JE et al. (1975) Respiratory care warrants studies for cost-effectiveness. Hospital 49(22): 61–71.

Calverley P, Belamy D (2000) The challenge of providing better care for patients with chronic obstructive pulmonary disease: the poor relation of airways obstruction. Thorax 55(1): 78–82.

Foglio K, Bianchi L, Bruletti G et al. (1999) Long-term effectiveness of pulmonary rehabilitation in patients with chronic airway obstruction. European Respiratory Journal 13(1): 125–132.

Goldstein RS, Gort EH, Stubbing D et al. (1994) Randomised controlled trial of respiratory rehabilitation (comment). Lancet 344(8934): 1394–1397.

Goldstein RS, Gort EH, Guyatt GH et al. (1997) Economic analysis of respiratory rehabilitation. Chest 112(2): 370–379.

Griffiths TL, Burr ML, Campbell IA et al. (2000) Results at 1 year of outpatient multidisciplinary pulmonary rehabilitation: a randomised controlled trial. Lancet 355(9201): 362–368.

Griffiths TL, Phillips CJ, Davies S et al. (2001) Cost effectiveness of an outpatient multidisciplinary pulmonary rehabilitation programme. Thorax 56(10): 779–84.

Guyatt GH, Berman LB, Townsend M et al. (1987) A measure of quality of life for clinical trials in chronic lung disease. Thorax 42(10): 773–778.

Haggerty MC, Stockdale-Woolley R, Nair S (1991) Respi-Care: an innovative home care program for the patient with chronic obstructive pulmonary disease. Chest 100(3): 607–612.

Holle RHO, Williams DV, Vandree JC et al. (1988) Increased muscle efficiency and sustained benefits in an outpatient community hospital-based pulmonary rehabilitation program. Chest 94(6): 1161–1168.

Hudson LD, Tyler ML, Petty TL (1976) Hospitalization needs during an outpatient rehabilitation program for severe chronic airway obstruction. Chest 70(5): 606–610.

Petty TL, Nett LM, Finigan MM et al. (1969) A comprehensive care program for chronic airway obstruction. Methods and preliminary evaluation of symptomatic and functional improvement. Annals of Internal Medicine 70(6): 1109–1120.

Reina-Rosenbaum R, Bach JR, Penek J (1997) The cost/benefits of outpatient-based pulmonary rehabilitation. Archives of Physical Medicine and Rehabilitation 78(3): 240–244.

Ries AL, Kaplan RM, Limberg TM et al. (1995) Effects of pulmonary rehabilitation on physiologic and psychosocial outcomes in patients with chronic obstructive pulmonary disease. Annals of Internal Medicine 122(11): 823–832.

Roselle S, D'Amico FJ (1982) The effect of home respiratory therapy on hospital readmission rates of patients with chronic obstructive pulmonary disease. Respiratory Care 27(10): 1194–1199.

Singh SJ, Smith DL, Hyland ME et al. (1998) A short outpatient pulmonary rehabilitation programme: immediate and longer-term effects on exercise performance and quality of life. Respiratory Medicine 92(9): 1146–1154.

Troosters T, Gosselink R, Decramer M (2000) Short- and long-term effects of outpatient rehabilitation in patients with chronic obstructive pulmonary disease: a randomized trial. American Journal of Medicine 109(3): 207–212.

White RJ, Rudkin ST, Ashley J et al. (1997) Outpatient pulmonary rehabilitation in severe chronic obstructive pulmonary disease. Journal of the Royal College of Physicians of London 31(5): 541–545.

Wijkstra PJ, Strijbos JH, Koeter GH (2000) Home-based rehabilitation for patients with COPD: organization, effects and financial implications. Monaldi Archives for Chest Disease 55(2): 130–134.

Wijkstra PJ, Ten Vergert EM, van Altena R et al. (1995) Long-term benefits of rehabilitation at home on quality of life and exercise tolerance in patients with chronic obstructive pulmonary disease. Thorax 50(8): 824–828.

Wijkstra PJ, van der Mark TW, Kraan J et al. (1996) Long-term effects of home rehabilitation on physical performance in chronic obstructive pulmonary disease. American Journal of Respiratory and Critical Care Medicine 153(4 part 1): 1234–1241.

Chapter 12
Future prospects for pulmonary rehabilitation

P. M. A. CALVERLEY

Introduction

As the other chapters in this book have amply demonstrated, there is now a wealth of evidence-based practice in the field of pulmonary rehabilitation. There can no longer be any significant doubt about the benefits of pulmonary rehabilitation in diseases like chronic obstructive pulmonary disease (COPD). This view is supported by carefully conducted meta-analysis of existing papers (Anon 1997, Lacasse et al. 1996) and has been accepted by all the major groups that have formulated treatment guidelines, including the Global Initiative for Chronic Obstructive Lung Disease (Pauwels et al. 2001). The striking thing for those unfamiliar with this field is the magnitude of the improvements seen, and those patients who successfully complete a rehabilitation programme are frequently amongst the most grateful we meet in clinical practice. Having achieved this rather belated breakthrough in terms of acceptance by the medical community, it would now seem sensible to consider what the next tasks should be if the potential of pulmonary rehabilitation is to be fully realized.

The slow uptake of pulmonary rehabilitation in the past could be seen as a consequence of asking the wrong questions in the wrong way. Thus the failure to demonstrate any improvement in lung function led many clinicians to underestimate the real impact of this important therapy. When considering future developments, it is important that there should be a clear hypothesis that is tested with robust tools in carefully conducted clinical trials. The present widespread acceptance of the value of pulmonary rehabilitation has been based on steps such as this, and enthusiasm for new developments must be tempered by the acquisition of evidence that is at least as good as that which we already have. The encouraging thing now is that there are many areas of active research in the field of pulmonary rehabilitation, and this chapter will inevitably be selective in focusing on some of those that appear to hold most promise. Progress is likely to result from a combination of increased knowledge of the underlying mechanisms that either limit the patient in their daily activities or limit their uptake of effective therapy. This, coupled with developing new treatment approaches, is the most probable way in which more effective rehabilitation strategies will be developed.

Studies in basic science

The impact of pulmonary rehabilitation on the patient is global and multi-dimensional, and so it can be hard to specify a single discipline on which basic scientific knowledge must be focused. The bulk of evidence, particularly from patients with COPD, has stressed that the benefits of rehabilitation are related to the exercise component of the regime (Barnes 1998), and understandably much scientific endeavour has gone into explaining why exercise is limited in patients in the first place. Three important areas have emerged.

Limits to muscle performance

Studies of muscle biopsies of patients at rest have indicated changes in the fibre type of the skeletal muscle together with reductions in the oxidative enzymes necessary for the generation of high-energy phosphates during exercise (Maltais et al. 1996, Maltais et al. 1999, Maltais et al. 2000, Pouw et al. 1998). Reductions in limb muscle force generation, especially in patients treated with oral corticosteroids, have been related to health utilization and mortality (Decramer et al. 1994, 1997). Reductions in body mass index and lean body mass have also been related to adverse health outcomes (Schols et al. 1998) and the fact that upper- as well as lower-limb muscles have been involved has strengthened the view that a specific skeletal muscle myopathy accompanies conditions such as COPD and explains the physiological impairment in this setting. Although markers of systemic inflammation have been found in such patients and been related to muscle strength (Schols et al. 1999), the magnitude of the changes seen appears to be relatively modest compared to other pulmonary disorders with a systemic component, e.g. bronchiectasis. Thus the systemic component in this disease is likely to be playing a role but is unlikely to be the only explanation of impaired exercise capacity.

More recently, there has been a revival of interest in the problems of oxygen delivery to exercising muscles in both cardiac and respiratory disease. Studies of the number of capillaries in these muscles, as well as calculations of oxygen diffusion distance, suggest that these features, involved in oxygen delivery to exercising muscles, are impaired in COPD (Jobin et al., 1998). More recently, studies in normal individuals have suggested that impaired cardiac output can occur even in healthy subjects who develop high intra-thoracic pressures when breathing through a Starling resistor. Although an imperfect model of the changes in lung mechanics in obstructive lung disease, this does emphasize that there are many reasons for impaired oxygen delivery during exercise, and, taken together with the impairment in muscle metabolic activities already reported, it is no surprise that these patients have low anaerobic thresholds as well as being limited in their exercise capacity by leg fatigue.

There are already some interesting studies using magnetic resonance spectoscopy that have confirmed the benefits of rehabilitation on intracellular pH (Sala et al. 1999). Newer techniques that permit the direct measurement of blood supply during exercise can readily be coupled to these established techniques and should offer a more precise explanation for the limitation of muscle performance during exercise.

Limitations on pulmonary performance

Most work in this area is being conducted in patients with COPD, and again new technologies changing our understanding of the limitations to exercise in these subjects are being developed. Most investigators attribute limited pulmonary performance to impaired lung mechanics and specifically the development of expiratory flow limitation during tidal breathing. This can be detected at rest, non-invasively, using the negative expiratory pressure technique, although more recent work in our own laboratory suggests that this can also be done reliably by measuring the change in impedance between inspiration and expiration. Recent studies have suggested that some patients are limited by dynamic hyperinflation, which occurs when the expiratory time is too short for the patient to reach the true elastic equilibrium volume, and as a result they begin to breathe at levels above this point. Dynamic hyperinflation tends to be progressive in COPD and is related to the intensity of breathlessness.

Detailed studies of the relationship of this phenomenon to flow limitation are so far not being performed, although, in general, patients who exhibit tidal flow limitation at rest are much more likely to show dynamic hyperinflation, and this can be monitored, with practice, using the inspiratory capacity method. In contrast, individuals without this tend to have a larger inspiratory reserve volume but are still limited in their exercise performance, possibly by impaired peripheral muscle function. Understanding the differences between flow-limited and non-flow-limited individuals is clearly going to be important if appropriate individual rehabilitation strategies are to be constructed. This aspect of lung mechanics has predominated in recent years over the earlier interest in simply increasing respiratory muscle strength. There is a general feeling that respiratory muscle training is beneficial, although it has proven harder to demonstrate this conclusively. Indeed, general strength training for all skeletal muscle has not been particularly effective in increasing exercise capacity, at least as assessed in the exercise laboratory. This rather surprising finding needs further investigation.

Limits to daily activities

To date, little attention has been paid to the factors that determine how much of an individual's exercise capacity is actually used in their daily lives. The general assumption is that people exercise maximally throughout the day, but preliminary data based on home-activity monitors suggest a more complex picture of significant variation with age, and individuals adopting different strategies at different times. Clearly, the tasks to be completed will vary, depending on the individual's home circumstance, possibly explaining why those who are socially isolated often find coping at home a much more difficult task. Home-activity monitoring offers a potentially useful approach to quantifying these otherwise subjective statements, and relating changes in daily activity recorded in the laboratory in more formal circumstances to those actually undertaken at home. Approaches of this kind may help to explain why the substantial gain experienced by most patients at the end of rehabilitation is not maintained more effectively, even in those who appear to be attending for regular maintenance sessions. Whether characteristic patterns of home performance exist in patients who experience common co-morbidities, such as depression, remains to be established, but at least new tools are being made available that may aid the understanding of these potentially important processes.

New therapeutic approaches

New therapeutic approaches have been developed which show promise as adjuncts to rehabilitation. Three general types of therapy are worth considering:

Electrical stimulation of muscles

Although at first reminiscent of the wider claims of the fringe medicine and diet community, there is clear scientific evidence that muscles that undergo regular electrical stimulation can increase their force, and this can translate into worthwhile improvements in exercise performance. To date, this approach has been studied most scientifically by workers in Glasgow, but it is hoped that the techniques that they have developed can be applied in other circumstances. The idea of increasing people's muscle strength in an involuntary fashion has considerable appeal as a way of addressing the concerns of those patients who are less able initially to participate in rehabilitation, or perhaps are less motivated and who need evidence that they can improve to believe that working at this is possible. Defining the optimum frequency, stimulation pattern and duration are clearly challenging issues for the coming years; whether other barriers such as the prior nutritional state of the patient will limit this approach remains to be determined, but it is one of the more innovative and attractive ideas to come into the field of pulmonary rehabilitation in the past few years.

Neutriceuticals

Exercise physiology and sports medicine have been aware for a number of years of the practice, widespread amongst performance athletes, of taking nutritional supplements to try to increase exercise capacity. Initial studies using androgens, either nandrolene, deconate or testosterone, in patients with COPD have been disappointing. While it has been possible to increase muscle strength in the short term, this is not translated into improved exercise capacity, at least as evaluated by endurance exercise testing. However, there is now an increasing theoretical argument for the use of nutritional supplements such as creatine, which is available at most health-food shops and has been shown to be taken up during regular dosing in healthy individuals by the major muscle groups. Theoretically, this should allow more high-energy phosphate to be available within the muscle and hence increase endurance. In practice, in healthy subjects during chronic dosing this has not proved to be the case. Whether the same would be true in patients with the complex metabolic limitations seen in COPD is another matter entirely, and several groups are beginning to test the validity of this treatment approach. Inevitably, other trace elements are being combined with natural muscle product, and further studies will be required to determine whether these other potentially valuable combinations have a role in the routine management of patients undergoing pulmonary rehabilitation.

Unloading ventilation

Studies using short- and long-acting inhaled bronchodilator drugs have indicated that, in COPD, ventilatory limitation is the commonest reason for stopping exercise. Effective drug therapy has increased the number of patients who are restricted by leg fatigue, a symptom which can be potentially improved by rehabilitation. This is part of the justification for multimodality therapy in this condition. Other ways of reducing the mechanical burden placed on the respiratory system are now being explored. These include the use of reduced-density gas mixtures of helium and oxygen, as well as having patients exercise while breathing with pressure-support ventilation. Data using the latter technique have been published and suggest that exercise capacity can be improved with this therapy. It may be possible to increase the intensity of exercise training if patients are supported in this way, and potentially to reduce the metabolic demands from exercising muscle on patients who are otherwise limited by their severely impaired lung mechanics. It has been suggested that giving supplementary oxygen during exercise has this effect already, and whether these different mechanisms can be usefully combined has not yet been fully tested. The role of supplementary oxygen in rehabilitation remains controversial, with no definite advantage for those who have undergone rehabilitation with oxygen compared with those without. However, this is a contentious area that is likely to be revisited in future.

Practical issues

In addition to the basic science and new modalities that research in rehabilitation has stimulated, there are still many practical issues that require resolution. In many health care systems, the availability of rehabilitation is limited and hence optimizing the period during which patients attend courses is an important consideration. Most courses are conducted on an outpatient basis, although some more affluent facilities can afford to hospitalize patients for six weeks of intensive therapy. Initial data comparing short courses of intensive in-patient hospitalization in conventional outpatient therapy suggest the latter is superior, while previous studies have indicated that, in most patients, outpatient therapy is as effective as inpatient care. Clearly there are issues here of selection bias and patient motivation, and certainly no definitive data yet available on the best duration and intensity of courses. Similarly, differences in the type of exercise test used to evaluate patients, and hence assess the effectiveness of therapy, have not yet been fully quantified. There are remarkably few studies comparing exercise capacity measured in the laboratory with field tests, such as corridor walking distance and shuttle walking tests, and it is likely that each gives somewhat different perspectives on the disability experienced by the patients.

Ultimately, the greatest problem remains the issue of optimal maintenance care. Whether this is a problem wholly related to declining participation in home exercise, as proposed above, or represents a genuine physiological regression to the mean, is unknown. Encouraging new data from Canada are expected to emerge showing that important health care gains can be made if people participate in an extended care programme following rehabilitation. However, the applicability of this to other health care systems has not yet been evaluated. Identifying better strategies for the significant numbers of people who do not wish to, or are unable to, participate in pulmonary rehabilitation programmes is going to be a key task for future effective management.

Conclusion

As we enter a new century, it is appropriate to feel optimistic about the impact of pulmonary rehabilitation on patient health. As with all effective treatments, its current successes have highlighted new problems that must be addressed, and new challenges that must be met. Regrettably, funding for these important practical issues is often difficult to obtain, but, despite that, the research within the clinical community in this area has every reason to view the future positively, an attitude which, it is to be hoped, can be conveyed to their patients.

References

Anonymous (1997) Pulmonary rehabilitation: joint ACCP/AACVPR evidence-based guidelines. ACCP/AACVPR Pulmonary Rehabilitation Guidelines Panel. American College of Chest Physicians. American Association of Cardiovascular and Pulmonary Rehabilitation. Chest 112(5): 1363–1396.

Barnes PJ (1998) Anti-inflammatory actions of glucocorticoids: molecular mechanisms. Clinical Science 94(6): 557–572.

Decramer M, Gosselink R, Troosters T et al. (1997) Muscle weakness is related to utilization of health care resources in COPD patients. European Respiratory Journal 10(2): 417–423.

Decramer M, Lacquet LM, Fagard R et al. (1994) Corticosteroids contribute to muscle weakness in chronic airflow obstruction. American Journal of Respiratory and Critical Care Medicine 150(1): 11–16.

Jobin J, Maltais F, Doyon JF et al. (1998) Chronic obstructive pulmonary disease: capillarity and fiber-type characteristics of skeletal muscle. Journal of Cardiopulmonary Rehabilitation 18(6): 432–437.

Lacasse Y, Wong E, Guyatt GH et al. (1996) Meta-analysis of respiratory rehabilitation in chronic obstructive pulmonary disease. Lancet 348(9035): 1115–1119.

Maltais F, Simard AA, Simard C et al. (1996) Oxidative capacity of the skeletal muscle and lactic acid kinetics during exercise in normal subjects and in patients with COPD. American Journal of Respiratory and Critical Care Medicine 153(1): 288–293.

Maltais F, Sullivan MJ, LeBlanc P et al. (1999) Altered expression of myosin heavy chain in the vastus lateralis muscle in patients with COPD. European Respiratory Journal 13(4): 850–854.

Maltais F, LeBlanc P, Whittom F et al. (2000) Oxidative enzyme activities of the vastus lateralis muscle and the functional status in patients with COPD. Thorax 55(10): 848–853.

Pauwels RA, Buist AS, Calverley PMA et al. (2001) Global strategy for the diagnosis, management and prevention of chronic obstructive pulmonary disease. American Journal of Respiratory and Critical Care Medicine 163(5): 1256–1276.

Pouw EM, Schols AM, Wouters EF et al. (1998) Elevated inosine monophosphate levels in resting muscle of patients with stable chronic obstructive pulmonary disease. American Journal of Respiratory and Critical Care Medicine 157(2): 453–457.

Sala E, Roca J, Marrades RM et al. (1999) Effects of endurance training on skeletal muscle bioenergetics in chronic obstructive pulmonary disease. American Journal of Respiratory and Critical Care Medicine 159(6): 1726–1734.

Schols AM, Creutzberg EC, Buurman WA et al. (1999) Plasma leptin is related to proinflammatory status and dietary intake in patients with chronic obstructive pulmonary disease. American Journal of Respiratory and Critical Care Medicine 160(4): 1220–1226.

Schols AM, Slangen J, Volovics L et al. (1998) Weight loss is a reversible factor in the prognosis of chronic obstructive pulmonary disease. American Journal of Respiratory and Critical Care Medicine 157(6 Part 1): 1791–1797.

Index

abdominal (diaphragmatic) breathing, 138–140
abdominal exercise, 43
activities of daily living (ADLs)
  breathlessness, 103
  future investigations, 190
  occupational therapy, 114, 115–123, 124
    assessment, 115–116, 118–119, 130–134
    economy of movement and effort, 120–123
    goal setting, 117–118
    patient profile, 115–116
    practical application, 120
    stress management and relaxation, 125, 126
    pacing, 85–86
activity monitors, 190
aerobic metabolism, 37, 38, 159–160
Age Concern, 109
age factors
  biopsychosocial approach, 79
  respiratory muscle endurance testing, 69
  selection for pulmonary rehabilitation, 17, 18
aims of pulmonary rehabilitation, 6
airflow obstruction
  asthma, 46, 47
  body function and structure, 4, 5
  breathing retraining, 139
  exercise limitation, 61
  exercise training, 37, 39, 46, 47
  nutritional depletion, 154
  physiotherapy, 139

selection for pulmonary rehabilitation, 11, 16, 18, 19
Airways Questionnaire 20 (AQ20), 32
American College of Chest Physicians, 2
anaerobic metabolism, 37, 38, 159–160
anthropometry, 156
antibiotics, 99, 102
anticholinergics, 98, 99, 107
antihypertensives, 107
anxiety
  aims of pulmonary rehabilitation, 6
  biopsychosocial approach, 79–80, 81, 83, 84, 87–93
  cognitive-behavioural programme, 84
  goal-setting, 118
  home-based care, 104
  measures, 83
  occupational therapy, 118, 124, 129
  palliative care, 109
  stress management and relaxation, 124, 129
  see also depression
appetite, 160–161, 166
AQ20 (Airways Questionnaire 20), 32
arm circling, 43
arm exercises, 39–40, 43–44
arm muscle area (AMA), 155
arm muscle testing, 62
arterial oxygen saturation, 160
arthritis, 18, 131
assessment process
  activities of daily living, 115–116, 118–119, 130–134
  biopsychosocial approach, 81–83
  exercise testing, 54–59

home-based care, 97, 103
measurements, 59–62
multidisciplinary team approach, 8
muscle function, 54–55, 62–69
nutritional status, 155–157, 165–166
occupational therapy, 103, 115–116,
  118–119, 130–134
asthma
  Airways Questionnaire 20 (AQ20), 32
  breathing retraining, 140–141
  cost-effectiveness of pulmonary
    rehabilitation, 179
  exercise-induced, 47, 55
  exercise testing, 55
  exercise training, 46–48
  home-based care, 96
  hyperventilation, 140
  physiotherapy, 140–141
attitude, see motivation and attitude

BBT (Buteyko Breathing Technique),
  140–141
BCM (body cell mass), 155, 156
bench press, supine, 42
benefits system, 109
Benzodiazepines, 109
beta-2 agonists
  Buteyko Breathing Technique trial,
    140–141
  exercise-induced asthma, 47
  home-based care, 98–99
  resting energy expenditure, 158
bicycle aerometry, 59
bicycle endurance test, 57
bicycle ergometer
  testing, 58
  training, 39, 40
bioelectrical impedance analysis (BIA),
  155–156
biofeedback, 90
biopsychosocial approach, 78–80,
  81–82, 94
  anxiety, 81, 87–93
  cognitive-behavioural programme,
    84–86
  components, 82–83
  depression, 80–81, 87–93
  goal-setting, 86–87
  measures, 83–84
  smoking cessation, 93–94, 98
  see also psychosocial issues and
    support

bisphosphonates, 100
blood supply, measurement during
  exercise, 189
Blue Badges, 109
BMD (bone mineral density), 157
BMI, see body mass index
body cell mass (BCM), 155, 156
body composition analysis, 155–157
body function and structure, 4–5
body mass index (BMI)
  equation, 105, 154
  and nutritional support, 165
  as prognostic factor, 154
body weight, see weight, body
bone mineral density (BMD), 157
Borg Breathlessness Scale (BBS), 139,
  143
  exercise testing, 59
  exercise training, 39, 41
Borg Symptom Scale, 56, 62
break-test, 64
Breathe Easy groups, 109
breathing exercises, 5, 44
  see also breathing techniques
Breathing Problems Questionnaire
  (BPQ), 24, 29
  effects of pulmonary rehabilitation, 30
  modification for clinical practice, 32
breathing techniques
  Buteyko Breathing Technique (BBT),
    140–141
  diaphragmatic breathing, 138–140
  hyperventilation management, 140
  occupational therapy, 120, 122,
    125–129
  physiotherapy, 138–143
  positioning, 142–143
  pursed-lips breathing, 142
  relaxation techniques, 141–142
  stress management and relaxation,
    125–129, 141–142
breathlessness
  activities of daily living, 116–117, 119,
    120, 131–132, 134
  anxiety and depression, 104–105
  asthma, 47, 48
  biopsychosocial approach, 79, 80, 85,
    86, 89
  dynamic hyperinflation, 189
  exacerbations, 102
  exercise testing, 57
  exercise training, 37, 39, 41, 44, 47, 48

goal-setting, 86
health-related quality of life, 23
home-based care, 98–100, 102,
    104–105
hyperinflation, 4, 189
medication, 98–100, 102
neuromuscular electrical
    stimulation, 146
occupational therapy 123, 124, 129
    activities of daily living, 116–117,
        119, 120, 131–132, 134
pacing, 85, 86
palliative care, 109
physiotherapy, 139–140, 142, 146
relaxation techniques, 124, 129
respiratory muscle training, 44
and sexuality, 106
stress management, 124, 129
see also dyspnoea
bronchiectasis, 188
bronchodilators, 98, 146, 158
bupropion, 98
Buteyko Breathing Technique (BBT),
    140–141

calcitonin, 100
calcium, 100
calf exercises, 42, 43
calf raises, 42
Canadian Occupational Performance
    Measure (COPM), 133–134
carbohydrate, 161–162
cardiocirculatory limitation to exercise,
    60, 61
cardiopulmonary resuscitation
    facilities, 49
cardiovascular disease, 18
carers, see families and carers
catastrophizing thoughts, 87, 88–89, 90
change, model of, 93–94
characteristics of rehabilitation
    programmes, 5–6
chest physiotherapy, 18
chlorpromazine, 37
chronic obstructive pulmonary disease
    (COPD)
    activity limitation, 5
    biopsychosocial approach, 78–80,
        81–83, 94
        anxiety, 81, 87–93
        cognitive-behavioural programme,
            84–86

depression, 80–81, 87–93
        goal-setting, 86–87
        measures, 83–84
        smoking cessation, 93–94
    body function and structure, 4–5
    cost-effectiveness of pulmonary
        rehabilitation, 173, 175, 179
    dietary management, 154, 167
        assessment of nutritional status,
            155–157
        education, 167
        energy balance, 157–160
        nutritional intervention, 105–106,
            161–163
        outcome, 163–167
        reduced dietary intake, 160–161
    exercise limitation, 61
    exercise testing, 54, 57
    future prospects for pulmonary reha-
        bilitation, 187, 188–189, 191
    health-related quality of life, 22, 23,
        28–32
    heterogeneity, 8
    home-based care, 96
        anxiety and depression, 103–105
        breathlessness, 103
        medication, 98, 99, 100–102
        nutrition, 105–106
        palliative care, 108–110
        psychosocial support, 108
        smoking cessation, 97
    multidisciplinary team approach, 8
    muscle testing, 54–55, 62, 63–64, 66,
        68–69
    occupational therapy
        activities of daily living, 115, 116,
            117, 118–121, 132–134
        extension of care, 123–124
        stress management and relaxation,
            129
    physiotherapy, 150
        adjuncts to pulmonary
            rehabilitation, 144, 146, 147, 148
        breathing retraining, 139, 142–143
    prevalence, 96
    selection for pulmonary rehabilitation,
        11–12, 14, 15–19
    sexuality, 106–108
chronic respiratory disease
    questionnaire (CRDQ), 12, 13, 14,
        24, 29
    and COPM, comparison between, 134

cost-effectiveness analysis, 182
effects of pulmonary rehabilitation,
    30, 31, 32
minimum clinical important
    difference, 28
non-invasive positive pressure
    ventilation, 144, 145
clinical psychology, 6
    see also psychosocial issues and
    support
cognitive-behavioural approach, 81, 84
    depression and anxiety, 87–93
    pacing, 84–86
    panic attacks, 141
cognitive diaries, 89–90
community rehabilitation services
    effectiveness, 7–8
    exercise training, 149
    multidisciplinary teams, 6, 7, 8, 143
Community Respiratory Resource Unit,
    123–124
co-morbidity
    activities of daily living, 115
    depression, 80
    future investigations, 190
    health-related quality of life, 30
    nutritional interventions, 106
    occupational therapy, 115
    physical deconditioning, 37
    and selection for pulmonary
        rehabilitation, 18
computer-assisted dynamometers, 65–66
concentrators, 100
concurrent validity of questionnaires, 27
content validity of questionnaires, 26
context of pulmonary rehabilitation, 1–2
COPD, see chronic obstructive
    pulmonary disease
COPD self-efficacy questionnaire, 84
coping strategies, 17
COPM (Canadian Occupational
    Performance Measure), 133–134
corticosteroids, 11, 17, 98
cost/benefit analysis, 174, 177–181
cost-effectiveness of pulmonary
    rehabilitation, 2, 173–174, 181–182, 184
    cost/benefit analysis, 174, 177–181
    cost/utility analysis, 14, 174, 182–184
    direct cost analysis, 174–1744
cost/utility analysis, 14, 174, 182–184
CRDQ, see chronic respiratory disease
    questionnaire

creatine supplements, 191
creatinine height index, 156–157
criterion validity of questionnaires, 27
critical power, 57
Cronbach's alpha, 25, 26
cycle aerometry, 59
cycle endurance test, 57
cycle ergometer
    testing, 58
    training, 39, 40
cystic fibrosis, 143

deconditioning, 11, 37
    anxiety, 80
    asthma, 46
    occupational therapy, 116, 124, 132
definitions of pulmonary rehabilitation, 2
deltoid muscle, 67
Dennison, Charles, 1
depression
    biopsychosocial approach, 80–81, 83,
        84, 87–93
    cognitive-behavioural programme, 84
    goal-setting, 118
    home-based care, 103–105
    measures, 83
    occupational therapy, 118
    recognition, 104–105
    sexual intimacy as antidote to, 106
diabetes, 90
diaphragmatic breathing, 138–140
diaphragmatic paresis, 69
dietary management, 154, 167
    assessment of nutritional status,
        155–157
    carbohydrate/fat, 161–162
    characteristics of rehabilitation
        programmes, 5
    education, 167
    energy balance, 157–160
    and exercise, 164–165
    home-based care, 105–106
    multidisciplinary team, 6, 166
    oral nutritional supplements,
        163–164, 191
    outcome, 163–167
    practical implementation, 165–167
    protein, 162–163
    reduced dietary intake, 160–161
    selection for pulmonary
        rehabilitation, 18
    timing of, 165

differential relaxation, 121, 129
dihydrocodeine, 109
direct cost analysis, 174–177
disease-specific measures of health
    status, 24–25, 28, 29
    activities of daily living, 117, 130–132,
        133, 134
doctors in the multidisciplinary team, 6
drug therapy, *see* medication
dual-energy x-ray absorptiometry (DXA),
    157
dynamic hyperinflation, 189
dynamometry, 63–64, 65–66
dyspnoea
    aims of pulmonary rehabilitation, 6
    biopsychosocial approach, 78
    body function and structure, 4
    characteristics of rehabilitation
        programmes, 5
    dietary management, 161, 162
    effects of pulmonary rehabilitation,
        12, 30
    exercise testing, 55, 56, 59
    exercise training, 37, 39, 44
    occupational therapy
        activities of daily living, 116, 118,
            122, 130–131
        stress management and relaxation,
            124, 125, 127
    physiotherapy, 138–150
        adjuncts to pulmonary
            rehabilitation, 144–148
        breathing retraining, 138–143
        mobility, 149
        neuromuscular electrical
            stimulation, 146
        respiratory muscle training and
            rehabilitation, 146–147
        sputum clearance, 143
        supplemental oxygen and
            rehabilitation, 147–148
    reduced dietary intake, 160
    respiratory muscle training, 44
    respiratory muscle weakness, 54
    selection for pulmonary rehabilitation,
        17, 18
    see also breathlessness

education
    of families and carers, 82, 91, 132
    of patients
        aims of pulmonary rehabilitation, 6

biopsychosocial approach, 87, 90
    characteristics of rehabilitation
        programmes, 5
    depression and anxiety, 87, 90
    home-based care, 97
    nutrition, 167
    occupational therapy, 120, 124
    selection for pulmonary
        rehabilitation, 18
elbow flexors, 67
electrical stimulation of muscles, 146,
    190–191
electroencephalographic synchronicity,
    37
end-of-life decisions, 110
endorphins, 37
endurance tests, 57
endurance training, 40–41, 42
    asthma, 46
    facilities, 49
    selection for pulmonary rehabilitation,
        18
    specificity, 39
energy
    balance, 157–160, 161, 165
    conservation, 120–123, 129, 131
ergometry, 55, 58
    training specificity, 39, 40
ergonomics, 120, 121
ergotherapy, 18
EUROQoL, 30
exacerbations
    breathing retraining, 139
    energy balance, 165
    home-based care, 100–102
    hospital referral criteria, 102
    occupational therapy, 124
    physiotherapy, 139
exercise
    commitment, 6, 120
    protocol, 58–59
    training (prescription), 4–5, 36–37
        assessment of performance, 54–62
        asthma, 46–48
        characteristics of rehabilitation
            programmes, 5
        dose response effect, 45–46
        effects of pulmonary rehabilitation, 14
        facilities, 48–49
        intensity, 37–38, 39
        low-intensity muscle group training,
            41–44

maintenance, 45–46
mobility, 149
multigym training, 40–41, 42–44
non-invasive positive pressure
  ventilation, 144
and nutritional interventions,
  164–165, 166
oxygen use, 48, 147–148
pursed-lips breathing, 142
respiratory muscle training, 44,
  146–147
reversibility, 44–45
selection for pulmonary
  rehabilitation, 18
specificity, 39–40
sputum clearance, 143
whole-body training, 37–40
tolerance/capacity, 11, 39, 54
aims of pulmonary rehabilitation,
  6, 12
asthma, 47
benefits of pulmonary
  rehabilitation, 14
breathing retraining, 139, 142
future investigations, 189, 190, 192
limiting factors, 59, 60–62
measurement, 59–60
neuromuscular electrical
  stimulation, 146
non-invasive positive pressure
  ventilation, 144, 145
nutritional interventions, 162
selection for pulmonary
  rehabilitation, 15
supplemental oxygen, 147
exercise-induced asthma (EIA), 47, 55
extracellular compartment, 155, 156

face validity of questionnaires, 26
factor analysis, 26
families and carers
biopsychosocial approach, 82, 91
home-based care, 98, 102, 108
occupational therapy, 123, 132
pacing, 123
palliative care, 110
recognition of role, 2
sexuality, 106, 107
smoking, 98
fat, dietary, 161–162
fat free mass (FFM), 155, 156–157
nutritional support, 165

protein metabolism, 162
and resting energy expenditure, 158
fatigue
activities of daily living, 120, 122, 131
breathing retraining, 140
effects of pulmonary rehabilitation, 12
exercise testing, 56, 57
leg, 4, 189, 191
occupational therapy, 120, 122, 125,
  126, 131
physiotherapy, 140
stress management and relaxation,
  125, 126
fat mass compartment (FMC), 155, 156
fear, 6, 118, 124
  see also anxiety
FFM, see fat free mass
field tests, 55–57
Flesch Formula, 81
flu vaccination, 99
FMC (fat mass compartment), 155, 156
forced expiratory volume in one second
  (FEV$_1$), 15–16, 18, 98, 116
free walking, 39, 40, 48
full-arm circling, 43
functional ability and training, 5, 6, 14
occupational therapy, 116, 133
Functional Independence Measure
  (FIM), 134
future prospects for pulmonary
  rehabilitation, 187–188, 192–193
new therapeutic approaches, 167,
  190–192
practical issues, 192
studies in basic science, 188–190

gender factors, 17
general practitioners, 14, 100
generic measures of health status,
  24–25, 28, 29
activities of daily living, 132–134
biopsychosocial approach, 83
goal-setting, 86
occupational therapy, 116, 117–118,
  130, 131, 132
rewards, 87
SMART, 86
smoking cessation, 116
group dynamics, 118

HAD (Hospital Anxiety and Depression)
  scale, 83

handgrip strength, 63–64
hand-held dynamometry, 63, 64–65
health-related quality of life (HRQoL)
    activities of daily living, 120
    benefits of pulmonary rehabilitation,
        12, 14
    benefits system, 109
    biopsychosocial approach, 79, 80
    breathing retraining, 140
    cost/utility analysis, 182–184
    definition, 22
    exercise training, 45–46
    goal-setting, 117
    vs. health status, 23
    home-based care, 96
    individualization vs. standardization,
        23–24
    measuring, 23, 27–28
    non-invasive positive pressure
        ventilation, 144, 145
    occupational therapy, 117, 120
    palliative care, 109, 110
    physiotherapy, 140
    and pulmonary rehabilitation, 28–32
    questionnaires
        design and development, 25
        generic vs. disease-specific, 24–25
        reliability, 25–26
        sensitivity, 27
        validity, 26–27
    reasons for measuring, 23
    research tool vs. clinical practice tool,
        32
    selection for pulmonary rehabilitation,
        19
    sexual problems, 106
    types of instrument, 28, 29
    use in clinical practice, 32–33
    see also health status
health status, 23
    see also health-related quality of life
heart rate, 38, 61
helium and oxygen mixtures, 191
holistic programme, rationale for, 3–4
home aids, 103, 120–124
home-based care, 96–97, 110
    anxiety and depression, 103–105
    assessment, 97
    breathlessness, 103
    cost/benefit analysis, 179
    exercise training, 7, 41, 45
    future investigations, 190

history, 97
    medication, 98–103
    neuromuscular electrical stimulation,
        146
    nutrition, 105–106
    occupational therapy, 123–124, 143
    palliative care, 108–110
    physiotherapy, 103, 143, 146, 149
    psychosocial support, 108
    sexuality, 106–108
    smoking cessation, 97–98
home helps, 103
hormone replacement, 100
hospice care, 102
Hospital Anxiety and Depression (HAD)
    scale, 83
hospital at home schemes, 102
hospital care
    effects of pulmonary rehabilitation on,
        14, 178, 179–80
    referrals to, 102–103
HRQoL, see health-related quality of life
HRQoLRIQ (Quality of Life in
    Respiratory Illness Questionnaire), 24
hypercapnia, 44, 54
hyperinflation, 4, 189
hypermetabolism, 157, 158–160
hyperventilation, 140, 141
hypoxemia, 61

immune system, 163
impotence, 107
increasing arm circles, 43
incremental exercise testing, 58
incremental shuttle walking test, 56–57
inflammation, 4, 18, 158–159, 160
influenza vaccination, 99
information leaflets, 81
information for patients, 90, 106, 107
    see also education
inhalers, 80, 99, 123, 124
inspiratory muscle training, 44
insulin-dependent diabetes, 90
intensive therapy units (ITUs), 110
interleukin 6 (IL-6), 18
interleukin 8 (IL-8), 18
internal consistency, quality of life
    questionnaires, 26
International Classification of Funding, 3
inter-observer agreement, quality of life
    questionnaires, 26
interval training, 18, 39

intracellular compartment (body cell
    mass), 155, 156
ischemic cardiovascular disease, 18
isometric muscle testing, 62, 63, 64–66
isotonic muscle testing, 65–66

Kappa statistic, 26
keyworker approach, 124

lactic acidosis, 4, 5, 16, 38
latissimus pull down, 42
leg curls, 42
leg extension, 42
leg fatigue, 4, 189, 191
leg muscle testing, 62
leg press, 42
leptin, 160–161
leukotrienes, 47
libido, 106, 107
life-saving procedures, 49, 56
living wills, 110
London Chest Activity of Daily Living
    Scale (LCADL), 132
long-term oxygen therapy (LTOT),
    100, 101
lower-limb training, 39, 40, 43–44
low-intensity muscle group training, 41–44
LTOT (long-term oxygen therapy), 100,
    101
lung-function technicians, 6
lung-function tests, 4
lung transplantation, 16, 18, 144
lung volume reduction surgery (LVRS)
    home-based preparation for, 7
    quality of life, 13
    selection for pulmonary rehabilitation,
        16, 18
    smoking cessation, 98

maintenance issues
    biopsychosocial approach, 92–93, 94
    exercise training, 45, 46
    future investigations, 192
    smoking cessation, 94
make-test, 64
malnourishment, 105
massage, 149
maximal exercise testing, 58–59
maximal expiratory mouth pressure,
    67–68, 69
maximal inspiratory mouth pressure,
    67–68, 69

maximal oxygen uptake, 59, 60
Medical Outcomes Study Short Form-36
    (MOS SF-36), 24, 29
    biopsychosocial approach, 83
    effects of pulmonary rehabilitation,
        30, 31
medication
    biopsychosocial approach, 80
    breathlessness, 109
    Buteyko Breathing Technique, 141
    compliance/concordance, 99
    home-based care, 98–103
    libido affected by, 107
    occupational therapy, 124
    over-the-counter, 99, 107
    and selection for pulmonary
        rehabilitation, 15
    side effects, 80
metabolic changes, 157–160
metered dose inhalers (MDIs), 99
minimum clinical important difference
    (MCID), 27–28
mobile phones, 103
mobility, 149
Modified Pulmonary Functional Status
    and Dyspnoea Questionnaire
    (PFSDQ-M), 131–132
Morriston Occupational Therapy
    Outcome Measure (MOTEM), 118
motivation and attitude
    biopsychosocial approach, 81, 86, 87,
        93
    exercise training, 46
    goal-setting, 86, 87, 118
    occupational therapy, 118, 123
    pacing, 123
    and selection for pulmonary
        rehabilitation, 17, 19
    smoking cessation, 93, 98
mucolytics, 99
multidisciplinary team, 6–8, 37
    biopsychosocial framework, 79
    home-based care, 97
    nutritional support, 6, 166
    occupational therapy, 6, 114, 123–124
    physiotherapy, 6, 141–142, 143, 148,
        149
multigym training, 40–41, 42–44, 48, 49
muscle endurance
    peripheral muscles, 6, 66–67
    respiratory muscles, 6, 44, 69
muscle strength/weakness, 4–5, 11

benefits of pulmonary rehabilitation, 14
peripheral muscles
  aims of pulmonary rehabilitation, 6
  benefits of pulmonary rehabilitation,
    14
  characteristics of rehabilitation
    programmes, 5
  electrical stimulation, 146, 190–191
  exercise limitation, 60, 61–62
  exercise training, 40, 42–44,
    146–147, 189
  limits to muscle performance,
    188–189
  neuromuscular electrical
    stimulation, 146
  nutrition, 164–165
  nutritional supplements, 191
  selection for pulmonary
    rehabilitation, 18
  testing, 54–55, 62–66, 69
respiratory muscles, 4
  aims of pulmonary rehabilitation, 6
  exercise limitation, 61
  exercise training, 5, 44, 146–147,
    189
  nutrition, 164
  testing, 54–55, 62, 67–69

National Health Service Research and
  Development Directorate, 2
National Institutes of Health (NIH), 2
NEADL (Nottingham Extended ADLs
  Scale), 133
nebulizers, 80, 99
negative automatic thoughts (NATs), 87,
  88–89
neuromuscular disease, 69
neuromuscular electrical stimulation
  (NMES), 146, 190–191
neutriceuticals, 167, 191
nicotine-replacement therapy, 98
Nijmegen Questionnaire, 141
nocturnal oxygen desaturation, 54
non-invasive positive pressure
  ventilation (NIPPV), 5, 110, 144–145
Nottingham Extended ADLs Scale
  (NEADL), 133
Nottingham Health Profile, 29
number need to treat (NNT), 181–182
nutritional interventions, see dietary
  management
nutritional supplements, 163–164, 191

occupational therapy (OT), 114–115
  activities of daily living, 115–123
  assessment and outcome measures,
    130–134
  extension of care, 123–124
  home-based care, 103, 143
  multidisciplinary team, 6, 114,
    123–124
  stress management and relaxation,
    124–129
one-repetition maximum (1-RM)
  weightlifting, 63
opioids, 109
oral nutritional supplements, 163–164,
  191
osteoarthritis, 131
osteoporosis, 99–100, 131
OT, see occupational therapy
overactivity/underactivity cycle, 84–85
over-the-counter medication, 99, 107
oxygen, supplementary
  characteristics of rehabilitation
    programmes, 5
  in exercise training, 48
  future investigations, 191–192
  home-based care, 100, 101
  long-term oxygen therapy (LTOT),
    100, 101
  physiotherapy, 147–148
  smoking cessation, 98

pacing, 84–86, 122–123
palliative care, 108–110
panic
  biopsychosocial approach, 79
  cycle, 104
  goal-setting, 118
  occupational therapy, 118, 123, 124,
    126
  stress management and relaxation,
    124, 126, 141
panic alarms, 103
partners, see families and carers
passive smoking, 98
peripheral muscles
  endurance, 6, 66–67
  strength, see muscle strength/
    weakness, peripheral muscles
PFSDQ (Pulmonary Functional Status
  and Dyspnoea Questionnaire),
    130–131
  modified version (PFSDQ-M), 131–132

physiotherapy
　adjuncts to pulmonary rehabilitation,
　　144–148
　breathing retraining, 138–143
　dyspnoea, 138–150
　home-based care, 103, 143, 146, 149
　mobility, 149
　multidisciplinary team, 6, 141–142,
　　143, 148, 149
　neuromuscular electrical stimulation,
　　146
　respiratory muscle training and
　　rehabilitation, 146–147
　selection for pulmonary rehabilitation,
　　18
　sputum clearance, 143
　supplemental oxygen and
　　rehabilitation, 147–148
　see also exercise
PLB (pursed-lips breathing), 142
pneumococcal vaccination, 99
posture, 121, 125
power squats, 42
predictive validity of questionnaires, 27
primary care, 14, 100
protein, 162–163
psychosocial issues and support
　characteristics of rehabilitation
　　programmes, 5
　exercise limitation, 60, 62
　home-based care, 108
　multidisciplinary team, 6
　nebulizer use, 99
　selection for pulmonary rehabilitation,
　　18
　see also biopsychosocial approach
Pulmonary Functional Status and
　Dyspnoea Questionnaire (PFSDQ),
　　130–131
　modified version (PFSDQ-M), 131–132
pulmonary gas exchange limitation to
　exercise, 60, 61
pulmonary performance, limitations on,
　189
pulse oximetry, 100
pursed-lips breathing (PLB), 142

quadriceps, 4–5
　electrical stimulation, 146
　endurance testing, 67
　exercise capacity, 54
　exercise for, 43

Quality Adjusted Life Years (QALYs),
　14–15, 182–184
quality of life, see health-related quality
　of life; health status
Quality of Life in Respiratory Illness
　Questionnaire (HRQoLRIQ), 24
quality of well-being scale (QWS), 24, 29
　effects of pulmonary rehabilitation,
　　12, 30, 31

REE (resting energy expenditure),
　157–158, 159, 160
referrals to hospital, 102–103
relapse prevention, 92–93, 94
relaxation techniques, 90
　differential relaxation, 121, 129
　home-based care, 103
　occupational therapy, 124–129
　physiotherapy, 141–142
　sexuality, 106
reliability/repeatability of questionnaires,
　25–26
resistive loading, 44
respiratory muscles
　dyspnoea, 138–139, 143, 144
　endurance, 6, 44, 69
　strength, see muscle strength/
　　weakness, respiratory muscles
respiratory nurses, 6
respiratory technicians, 6
respite care, 102
resting energy expenditure (REE),
　157–158, 159, 160
resuscitation facilities, 49
rheumatoid arthritis, 18, 131

salbutamol, 158
Schedule for Evaluation of Individual
　Quality of Life (SEIHRQoL), 24
seating, 121, 122
selection for pulmonary rehabilitation
　programmes, 11–19
　benefits, 12–15
　biopsychosocial approach, 81–82
　exercise training, 62
self-efficacy, 78, 92, 93
self-management, 6, 14, 38, 41, 167
sensitivity of questionnaires, 27
settings for pulmonary rehabilitation, 7–8
sexuality, 106–108
SF36, see Medical Outcomes Study Short
　Form-36

SF-6D questionnaire, 183
SGRQ, *see* St George's Respiratory Questionnaire
shoulder shrugging, 43
shuttle running and walking tests, 55, 56–57
Sickness Impact Profile (SIP), 12–13, 24, 29
sitting position, and dyspnoea, 142–143
sit to stand exercise, 43
six-minute walking distance (6-MWD), 12, 13, 55–56
    training reversibility, 45
    training specificity, 39
skinfold thickness measurement, 155
sleeping patterns, 126
smoking, 78
    biopsychosocial approach, 82, 98
    cessation
        biopsychosocial approach, 82, 93–94
        home-based care, 97–98
        occupational therapy, 116
    and lung function, 11
    occupational therapy, 116
    and selection for pulmonary rehabilitation, 15
sniff manoeuvres, 69
social factors, 109
    see also psychosocial issues and support
social services, 6
somatic complaints, 109
spacers, 99
spirometry, 4
split-half reliability, 25
spouse, *see* families and carers
sputum clearance, 143
stair-lifts, 122
stairs, 143
step tests, 55
step-ups, 43–44
steroids, 98, 99–100, 107
St George's Respiratory Questionnaire (SGRQ), 24, 29
    biopsychosocial approach, 84
    effects of pulmonary rehabilitation, 12, 30, 31, 32
    minimum clinical important difference, 28
'STOP' relaxation technique, 127, 128, 129
storage within workspaces, 122

stress
    management, 115, 124–125, 126
    transactional model, 132
sub-maximal exercise testing, 55–57
substrate metabolism, 157–160
supine bench press, 42
supplementary oxygen, *see* oxygen, supplementary
survival rates, 14
sustainable pressure, 69

test–retest reliability, 25
Theophylline derivatives, 98, 107
threshold loading, 44
timed walking tests, 12, 13, 55–56
    training reversibility, 45
    training specificity, 39
time-out in group programmes, 91–92
total daily energy expenditure (TDE), 157, 159–160
transactional model of stress, 132
transitional dyspnoea index, 12
treadmill exercise, 40, 45, 47
treadmill tests, 58
triceps, 67
tumour necrosing factor-alpha (TNF-α), 18, 158–159
twelve-minute walking distance (12-MWD), 15, 55–56
twitch stimulation, 66

unloading ventilation, 191–192
upper-limb training, 39–40, 43–44
upright rowing, 42
utility scales, 28

vaccination, 99
validity of questionnaires, 26–27
vastus lateralis, 5, 18
ventilatory limitation to exercise, 60, 61
ventilatory muscle training (VMT), 146
visual analogue scale (VAS), 39, 59, 143
visualization techniques, 127, 129
vitamin D, 100

walking
    aids, 149
    distance, 15, 54, 55–56
    free walking, 39, 40, 48
    timed tests, 12, 13, 55–56
        training reversibility, 45
        training specificity, 39

wall-press-ups, 43
weight, body, 154, 155
  loss, 154
    energy balance, 157–160
    home-based care, 105
    oral nutritional supplements, 163, 164
    practical implementation of nutritional support, 165
    reduced dietary intake, 160–161
    timing of nutritional support, 165

weight training, 40–41
whole-body training, 37–40
wishful thinking, 17
workrate in exercise training, 37–39
World Health Organization, 3

Printed in the United Kingdom
by Lightning Source UK Ltd.
119716UK00001B/80